Ethical Issues in Nursing

Peggy L. Chinn, RN, PhD, FAAN
Editor

A collection of articles from *Advances in Nursing Science*
and *Topics in Clinical Nursing*

AN ASPEN PUBLICATION®
Aspen Systems Corporation

1986

Rockville, Maryland
Royal Tunbridge Wells

Library of Congress Cataloging in Publication Data
Main entry under title:

Ethical issues in nursing.

"An Aspen publication."
"A collection of articles from Advances in nursing science and Topics in
clinical nursing.
Includes index.
1. Nursing ethics—Addresses, essays, lectures.
I. Chinn, Peggy L. II. ANS, Advances in nursing science. III. Topics in
clinical nursing. [DNLM: 1. Ethics, Nursing—collected works. WY 85 E84]
RT85.E8   1986   174'.2   85-22905
ISBN: 0-87189-275-8

Library of Congress Catalog Card Number: 85-22905
ISBN: 0-87189-275-8

Printed in the United States of America

1 2 3 4 5

Contents

Preface

The value of the study of ethics in nursing and health care has long been recognized. The growing body of nursing literature has consistently included writings on the specific ethical concerns of nurses. The selections in this book, originally published in *Advances in Nursing Science* and *Topics in Clinical Nursing,* related ethical concerns to nursing as a science and as a practice discipline. The essays present an overview of the theoretical and philosophical dimensions of ethics in nursing, with particular emphasis on ethical issues in nursing practice and education. The volume provides a single, ready reference for these important issues in ethics. Each of the articles is as timely today as when it was first printed, and the ideas will continue to be useful for students, educators, and practitioners in the years to come.

The opening articles address fundamental issues of ethics in nursing. From these general considerations, the focus moves to more specific issues of autonomy, privacy, and rights related to life and death. The concluding articles address specific teaching approaches related to ethics and value choices.

As human beings, we all face ethical choices. We subscribe to values that reflect the moral and ethical fibers of our lives. We behave in ways that reveal the essence of our ethics and the broader structure of our values. We make choices in our personal lives every day that mirror the complex ethical heritage we acquire from our families and cultures and the emerging convictions that we formulate within as we grow and develop. We live with internal ambivalence and inconsistencies, often without consciously acknowledging that they exist. Except in religious training, we have few specific and direct resources that provide a means of formally examining the ethical components of our lives.

We share this human condition with every other human being, whether that other person is a coworker, a client, a teacher, a patient, another health care worker, or a friend. As nurses, however, we face ethical dilemmas that are not commonly found in other fields. Sometimes a particular ethical issue is of concern to other disciplines as well, but the nature of our choices and our perspective on them are unique to our role as nurses. The complexity of our ethical dilemmas as nurses increases immensely with each new technological development. With the growing involvement of increasingly complex social and political networks, we can no longer enjoy the luxury of relying on our family heritage, our religious training, or our own sense of "right" and "wrong" to guide our actions in relation to nursing. It is imperative that we all—teachers, students, practitioners, scholars, and researchers—actively study ethical theory, understand the skills of ethical inquiry, and rely on the conclusions of nurse ethicists to guide the development of ethics that govern choices in the discipline.

The very nature of ethics is one of dilemmas. The articles in this book reflect contradictions, inconsistencies, and alternative views that are inherent in ethical issues. Some of the contradictions are named and described by the authors; others will be detected by the reader from one article to the next. The challenge for the reader is one of sorting, testing, and carefully considering all that is possible in the range of human response to difficult ethical problems.

Peggy L. Chinn, Editor

The Ethics of Caring

Barbara A. Carper, R.N., Ed.D.
Associate Professor and Chairman
Division of Medical Surgical Nursing
College of Nursing
Texas Woman's University
Dallas Center
Dallas, Texas

THERE IS a growing litany of criticism to which health care providers have been increasingly exposed. One criticism among these involves issues that should be of primary concern to all of us, for they are the central and unifying focus of all health care providers: the phenomenon of care, the caring process and caring consequences. The charge of dehumanization by health care providers and the resulting depersonalization of the patient/client strikes at our professional commitment to provide both competent and caring help to the maimed, the injured and the diseased.[1]

This basic dictum to be compassionate, humane and caring toward those for whom we provide care is most often expressed in the phrase "treat the person not merely the patient." To be concerned with the "whole person" and to practice with consideration and sensitivity for the integrity of the human self is basically an ethical injunction.[2] Caring, as a professional and personal value, is of central

1

importance in providing a normative standard which governs our action and our attitudes toward those for whom we care.

THE EROSION OF CARE

The two factors that seem most pertinent to the process of caring are specialization and the development of science and technology.

Specialization

The trend toward specialization and institutionalization in medicine, nursing and other allied health care professions has resulted in a bewildering division and subdivision of tasks and claims to expertise. The vast superstructure of our highly institutionalized bureaucracy is inherently depersonalizing. The individual easily becomes lost in the maze of rigid and uniform regulations applied to all with an impersonal and many times apathetic hand.

The social milieu of most large teaching hospitals and clinics reflect what Goldsborough characterizes as a "no care" society.[3] Patients are at the mercy of strangers whose roles they do not and may never understand, and unfamiliar machines and alien routines that seem totally out of step with their own habits. The patient "becomes just another patient, another disease, another medication order, another name on the daily operating room schedule. . . . He is required to discard his identity as a person and become a 'patient'."[3(p66)]

It is perhaps not an altogether unreasonable observation that "Few people have a hospital experience without feeling to some degree depersonalized and deprived of basic human rights and dignities."[4(p314)] The health care team approach has in many ways been a reasonable response to the rapidly proliferating science and technology in the health care field. It has become almost a necessity in diagnosis and treatment. On the positive side, it must be acknowledged that there are many people alive today that might not be if it were not for these specialists' teams. However, the emergence of teams has raised serious issues about the relationship between and among the various professional team members and the team's influence on the quality of care provided to the patient.

Perhaps a more serious concern related to the specialized team approach is the tendency to devalue the individual. The

---

The parceling out of the patient to various team members has undoubtedly contributed to the increasing fragmentation and impotence felt in any encounter with the health care system.

---

parceling out of the patient to various team members has undoubtedly contributed to the increasing fragmentation and impotence felt in any encounter with the health care system.

The Development of Science and Technology

The "spirit of the age," or *Zeitgeist* as the Germans call it, of the 20th century has been the scientific method and its visible, material product, technology. The discoveries of medical and biological science, and the resulting technological applications, are successes of which modern medicine is justly proud. There is little doubt that future discoveries are certain to extend even further our knowledge of humans as objects of science.

Yet beneath this justifiable pride of accomplishments, certain events conceived in these same scientific successes have created a disquietude. Health care providers are in danger of generalizing scientific and technical expertise into the realm of individual patients' values and beliefs. The exercise of authority by health professionals, conferred by the power of clinical science and technology, carries with it the frightening potential of overshadowing individuals, reducing them to objects or abstractions, and of becoming an instrument of tyranny—when untempered by a humanistic value system.[5] There is a clear and present danger—considering the possibilities of genetic manipulation, behavior control and organ transplantation—of a failure to make clear the distinction between what *is* and what *ought* to be. "We cannot," Pellegrino cautions, "use the awesome powers of medicine humanely without rethinking our idea and images of man, and the value and purposes of his existence."[5(p14)]

The delivery of health care, regardless of how competently the specific tasks are carried out in relation to a given patient, or how consistent with the latest scientific knowledge it is, is often perceived by the client as lacking the "poignant personally experienced feeling of being cared for."[6(p837)] The quality of care is something quite separate from outcome of treatment. What we have gained in our understanding of humans, biological and material

objects, is inversely accompanied by a diminishing identity and sense of self.

There is much in literature about this mixed blessing of science. The Frankenstein myth is a compelling metaphor that describes how scientific and technological success has reduced rather than enhanced our humanity. The story of Dr. Victor Frankenstein and the monster he created is, on the surface, a novel of tensely mounting horror. On a more profound level, it offers a searching inquiry into the human condition. Although a grotesque exaggeration, it reflects the author's philosophical concern about peoples' constant striving for knowledge and control over the forces of nature.

Working alone in his laboratory, Dr. Frankenstein, finding that "the minuteness of the parts" was a hindrance, resolves to make his creature "about eight feet in height and proportionally large."[7(p52)] As he works, he speculates that with his success "a new species would bless me its creator and source; many happy and excellent natures would owe their being to me. . . . I might in process of time . . . renew life where death had apparently devoted the body to corruption."[7(p52–53)] Yet when the dull yellow eyes of his creature open he is filled with disgust and horror. Frankenstein's tragedy was not his scientific triumph over nature, but his *failure to care* for what he had created. He was unable to recognize or experience the humanness of another's self.

THE PROCESS OF CARING

In a world in which there is a great deal of loneliness, pain, suffering, illness and tragedy, the need for care has become essential. Although the concept of curing is perhaps the dominant focus in health care, Leininger maintains that "caring acts and decisions make the crucial difference in effective curing consequences. Therefore, it is caring that is the most essential and critical ingredient to any curative process."[8(p2)]

With dominant emphasis on curing, most discussions of health care or quality of care neglect the concept of "caring." Dictionary definitions of caring include a sense of close or careful attention, a sense of watchful responsibility, custody or management, a feeling of love or liking. Sobel defines human caring as "that feeling of concern, regard, respect, one human being may have for another."[9(p2612)] Caring includes a component of self-respect or dignity. Gaylin argues that an impulse for caring is biologically programmed in human nature.[10] This caring impulse may be impaired or reinforced by environmental circumstance.

Mayeroff describes caring as "a process, a way of relating to someone that involves development ... in time through mutual trust and a deepening and qualitative transformation of the relationship."[11(p1)] The meaning of caring, he suggests, "is not to be confused with such meanings as wishing well, liking, comforting and maintaining ... it is not an isolated feeling or a momentary relationship. . . ."[11(p1)]

Mayeroff explores what he describes as a general pattern of caring. In a caring relationship a person or an idea is experienced both as an extension and as something separate from oneself. One experiences what is cared for as having a dignity and worth in its own right with potentialities and need for growth. Caring is the antithesis of possessing, manipulating or dominating, a process which requires devotion and trust. In any actual instance of caring there must be someone or something specific that is cared for. Caring cannot occur by sheer habit; nor can it occur in the abstract.[11]

Major Components of Caring

Mayeroff further examined the concept of caring by describing what he identified as eight essential ingredients.

Knowledge that is both general and specific is required, since caring is not simply a matter of good intentions or warm regards. Caring includes explicit and implicit knowledge, knowing that and knowing how, and direct and indirect knowledge.

Alternating rhythms is the moving back and forth between a narrower and a wider framework. It is being able to maintain or modify behavior according to variations in circumstance or perspective.

Patience is a kind of perceptive participation with the other in which there is a sense of the other's own time and style. Patience is contrasted with a passive waiting for something to happen.

Honesty is a positive, active confrontation and being open to oneself and to the other rather than a matter of *not* doing something, such as not deliberately deceiving others.

Trust involves the appreciation of the independent existence of the other. Trusting the other is to let go and includes an element of risk and a dose of courage. Trust in a caring relationship is not being

---

> *Humility, which is present in the caring process, involves continuous learning and an awareness of the uniqueness of each new situation regardless of how extensive one's previous experience has been.*

---

indiscriminate, either in one's own or in another's capacity and judgment.

Humility is present in the caring process in several ways. It involves continuous learning and an awareness of the uniqueness of each new situation regardless of how extensive one's previous experience has been. It includes an acceptance of dependence and an awareness of personal limitations.

Hope, as an expression of a present alive with possibilities and plenitude, is not to be confused with wishful thinking and unfounded expectations. Hope implies that there is or could be something that is worthy of commitment and that mitigates against despair.

Courage makes risk taking possible, which carries one beyond safety and security. But it is not blind. It is a courage informed by knowledge, by past experiences and by a trust in one's own and in another's ability to grow.[11]

Others have described caring in terms of commitment; a way of life which finds expression in the "therapeutic use of the self."[12] The committed, Clemence said, is one who accepts full responsibility for one's action and is willing to take risks, to face danger, to be a "witness" to life. Those who refuse commitment by becoming detached, calloused and cynical are "spectators" to life rather than "witnesses."[12] Commitment and a therapeutic use of self is not, she warns, to "be advised heedlessly, nor claimed lightly . . . [they] . . . can be achieved only at the cost of anxiety and suffering."[12(p505)] Commitment, as an ingredient of caring, Levine said, is "the willingness to enter with the patient that predicament which he cannot face alone as an expression of moral responsibility; the quality of the moral commitment is a measure of the nurse's excellence."[13(p845)]

"Therapeutic use of self" is what I have described elsewhere as the component of personal knowledge.[14] It requires what may be referred to as the sacrifice of form; the awareness that abstract and generalized categories describing common group behaviors and traits can never encompass or express the uniqueness of the individual. The perception of a patient as a person goes beyond categorical recognition; it involves an active gathering of details and scattered particulars into an experienced whole for the purpose of seeing what is there. It is this kind of perception that results in a unity between an action taken and results.

Key Issues Related to Caring

Specialization and the impact of science and technology have been identified as two major influences affecting the process and the act of caring within the health care system. These factors can further be associated with a few key issues which seem more closely identified with any discussion of the ethics of caring:

1. the nature of the health care provider-patient relationship;

2. informed consent;
3. determination of the quality of life; and
4. determination of ethical participation in decision-making.

These key issues will be discussed together.

Any relation between two people or groups carries with it a set of mutual expectations. Obviously, the relationship between the health professional and the patient or client entails several unique features that other human relationships do not share. The exact nature of these features is not always clear nor agreed upon by different authorities. However, few would disagree that specialization within the health care system, the team approach and the specialization of health care providers have irretrievably altered the environmental context in which these human relationships occur.

Veatch has identified and characterized several idealized models of the physician-patient relationship.[15] Starting with Veatch's basic characterizations, these models can be expanded to include all professional health care provider-client relationships.

THE ENGINEERING MODEL

In the "engineering model" the health professional assumes the rhetoric and guise of the popularly conceived image of the scientist. He deals only with facts, divorcing himself from all questions of ethics and value considerations in the decision-making process. The health care provider's role in this model is to completely and dispassionately present the facts to the patient, let the patient decide and then proceed to carry out those decisions.

This approach, at first glance, would seem to maximize the participation of the patient in the decision-making process and to more than satisfy the essential ingredient of honesty in the caring process. On closer inspection, however, the "engineering" approach to human relationships is logically impossible and ethically outrageous.[15] It is impossible to be value-free in situations where choices must be made daily which affect the quality of life. Each decision requires a value judgment as to what is significant and what is right. This approach is morally irresponsible and reduces humans to objects of science and collapses the category of what *ought to be* to mean nothing more than *what is possible.*

This frightening image of the impartial application of science to health care is addressed in a moving and sensitive book entitled *A Very Easy Death* by the French author Simone de Beauvoir. The book is concerned with the examination of the day-by-day tragedy of her mother's death following the discovery of inoperable cancer of the intestines. The author, reflecting on the surgeons who were responsible for her mother's medical care, felt a liking for Dr. P because he talked to her mother "as though she were a human being and he answered my questions willingly."[16(p61)] On the other hand, she and her sister did not get along with Dr. N at all. Dr. N was "infatuated with technique, and he had resuscitated maman with great zeal; but for him she was the subject of an interesting experiment and not a person. He frightened us."[16]

THE PRIESTLY MODEL

The "priestly model" characterizes the health professional in the other extreme. The role assumed here is frankly paternalistic; it removes the locus of decision making from the patient and places it in the hands of the health care professional. According to Veatch, the chief diagnostic sign of this approach is the "speaking-as-a" syndrome. "The problem," he said, "is one of generalization of expertise: transferring of expertise in the technical aspects of a subject to expertise in moral advice."[15(p6)]

The "priestly" health care provider is presumed to have competence in both areas by virtue of his specialized knowledge and experience. There is no apparent awareness of the need for humility and no indication of trust or confidence in the other. There is, in addition, another more subtle dimension to this model which enlarges the moral questions: the failure to appreciate one of the essential requirements of caring, the alternating rhythm of moving back and forth between the narrower ethical framework of the particular professional group and the broader set of societal ethical norms. "That there exists a wide chasm between the value systems of society and of the professional practitioner seems inherent in the conflicts that characterize issues of health care delivery,"[17(p63)] Levine observed. The scope and power of medical science which has grown with increasing knowledge is not sufficient reason to justify the vestment of authority about what constitutes "harm" and "good" in any particular group of individuals. Pellegrino reminds us that "In a matter so personal as health, the imposi-tion of one person's values over another's . . . is a moral injustice."[1(p1293)]

THE CONTRACTUAL MODEL

The "contractual model" is a nonlegalistic agreement between the professional and the client regarding general obligations and expected benefits for both parties. The basic obligations are governed by the norms of individual freedom, such as preservation of individual dignity, insofar as choice and control over one's body and quality of life contributes to that dignity. Honesty is an inherent requirement in terms of truth telling and promise keeping to make possible a truly informed, voluntary consent. There is a mutual trust even though it is recognized that there may not be a complete mutuality of value sharing. There is an acknowledgement by the patient that the professional practitioner has the requisite skill to make the technical decisions. There is an acknowledgement by the professional practitioner that technical decisions are governed by a prior shared decision-making process that respects each party's moral integrity. Undoubtedly, this is an idealized model that obviously very few health care professional-client relationships conform to. However, if there is at least an attempt to aim at this ideal model, patients would have available to them the best science and technology that can be employed in their behalf in a "caring" relationship.

LEARNING TO BE MORE HUMANE

How then can we as health care professionals learn to be more humane and authentically caring? Some have advocated a greater emphasis on the social sciences and the humanities within the formal professional educational experience. Currently there are several professional schools attempting to integrate humanistic studies into the more traditionally conceived formal professional curricula.[18] Certainly study in those disciplines which provide us with a broader and more representative understanding of the factual and imaginative dimensions of the human condition is of benefit. The error in this approach, Clouser said, is to expect that a study of the humanities will make a person more humane.[19]

The study of the humanities within the context of a professional program, however, does offer a unique opportunity to utilize the readily available experiential data which center on personal involvement of the practitioner with the specific concerns of the patient. The possibility of the cultivation of the imagination and of compassion in dealing with patients, that is, the coming to know the uniqueness of the individual, is enhanced through empathic acquaintance.[20,21]

A complete awareness of the meaning of another's life experience is never possible. But empathic understanding can extend our range of imagined possibilities. Empathy may be defined as the capacity for

---

A complete awareness of the meaning of another's life experience is never possible. But empathic understanding can extend our range of imagined possibilities.

---

participating in or vicariously experiencing another's feelings. It requires one to imaginatively take the role of another in order to understand and accurately predict that person's thoughts, feelings and actions.

Empathy is moderated by detachment in order to apprehend and abstract what one is attending to, and in this sense is objective.[14] It is an affective attribute in much the same way as Pellegrino describes compassion in that it is reflected in a genuine capacity to feel and "to share in the pain and anguish . . . an . . . understanding of what sickness means to another person, together with a readiness to help and to see the situation as the patient does."[1(p1289)] Empathy is not what is commonly understood as pity or sympathy, nor should it be confused with condescension or paternalism. The empathic person is able to perceive multiple possibilities of meaning simultaneously and has the capacity to "listen to feelings and moods, to nonverbal behavior, as well as to words."[22(p13)]

Caring is not readily, if at all, learned in a classroom or a formal course of study. Some acquaintance with the social sciences and the humanities may contribute to our understanding of the real and imaginative dimensions of human existence. But it will not necessarily result in a caring attitude. To be humane, sensitive and caring practitioners, we must believe in the dignity and worth of the person, and we must understand firmly the meaning of values, choices and priority systems within which values are expressed.[1] We need especially to critically examine our own personal value systems and to identify "specific clinical situations in which value questions influence the outcome for human beings seeking help."[1(p1293)]

For those of us who profess to "care" for those we serve it should be agreed that "the wholeness which is part of our aware-ness of ourselves is shared best with others when no act diminishes another person, and no moment of indifference leaves him with less of himself."[13(p849)]

REFERENCES

1. Pellegrino, E. D. "Educating the Humanist Physician." *JAMA* 227:11 (March 18, 1974) p. 1288–1294.
2. Zaner, R. M. "The Unanchored Leaf: Humanities and the Discipline of Care." *Texas Reports on Biology and Medicine* 32:1 (Spring 1974) p. 1–18.
3. Goldsborough, J. "Involvement." *AJN* 69:1 (January 1969) p. 66–68.
4. McWilliams, R. M. "The Balance of Caring." *AORN J* 24:2 (August 1976) p. 314–320.
5. Pellegrino, E. D. *Medicine and Philosophy: Some Notes on the Flirtation of Minerva and Aesculapius* (Philadelphia: Society for Health and Human Values 1974).
6. Menninger, W. W. "Caring as Part of Health Care Quality." *JAMA* 234:8 (November 24, 1975) p. 836–837.
7. Shelley, M. *Frankenstein.* (New York: New American Library 1965).
8. Leininger, M. "Caring: The Essence and Central Focus of Nursing" in *The Phenomenon of Caring: Part V.* American Nurses' Foundation, Nursing Research Report, 12:1 (February 1977) p. 2–14.
9. Sobel, D. "Human Caring." *AJN* 69:12 (December 1969) p. 2612–2613.
10. Gaylin, W. *Caring* (New York: Alfred A. Knopf 1976).
11. Mayeroff, M. *On Caring* (New York: Harper & Row 1972) p. 1.
12. Clemence, M. "Existentialism: A Philosophy of Commitment." *AJN* 66:3 (March 1969) p. 500–505.
13. Levine, M. "Nursing Ethics and the Ethical Nurse" *AJN* (May 1977) p. 845–849.
14. Carper, B A. "Fundamental Patterns of Knowing in Nursing." *ANS* 1:1 (October 1978) p. 13–23.
15. Veatch, R. M. "Models for Ethical Medicine in a Revolutionary Age." *Hastings Center Rep* 2:3 (June 1972) p. 5–7.
16. de Beauvoir, S. *A Very Easy Death* (New York: Warner Books 1973).
17. Levine, M. "On the Nursing Ethic and the Negative Command" in *Fostering Ethical Values During the Education of Health Professionals* (Chicago: University of Illinois at the Medical Center and the Society for Health and Human Values 1976) p. 63–69.
18. Institute on Human Values in Medicine. *Human Values Teaching Programs for Health Professionals* (Philadelphia: Society for Health and Human Values 1976).
19. Clouser, D. K. "Philosophy and Medicine: The Clinical Management of a Mixed Marriage" in *Proceedings 1st Session, Institute on Human Values in Medicine* (Philadelphia: Society for Health and Human Values 1972) p. 47–80.
20. Lee, V. "Empathy" in Rader, M., ed. *A Modern Book of Esthetics* 3rd ed. (New York: Holt, Rinehart and Winston 1960).
21. Lippo, T. "Empathy, Inner Imitation and Sense-Feelings" in Rader, M., ed. *A Modern Book of Esthetics* 3rd ed. (New York: Holt, Rinehart and Winston 1960).
22. Kramer, M. and Schmalenberg, C. "The First Job—A Proving Ground Basis for Empathy Development." *J Nurs Admin* 7:1 (1977) p. 12–20.

The Nurse as Advocate: A Philosophical Foundation for Nursing

Leah L. Curtin, R.N., M.S., M.A.
Director
National Center for Nursing Ethics
Cincinnati, Ohio

NURSES seem to be moving in the direction of the medical model with its emphasis on science, technology and cure. As individual nurses and as members of a profession we are seeking fundamental clarifications and asking radical questions. In partial reaction to this move toward the medical model we seem to be diverting to what is essentially a historical model of nursing with an emphasis on an intuitive approach. The answers that we reach, the direction that we choose will determine the future parameters of nursing.

Some sociologists have suggested that rather than developing as nursing professionals, professional nurses are evolving out of nursing! "Nursing will still be nursing, but it will be carried on by persons of other occupational affiliations."[1(p528)] What then will nurses be doing while someone else is doing nursing?

According to some nursing leaders, nurses will be moving on to "meta-nursing."[2] Travelbee claims that "The role of the nurse must be transcended in order to relate as human being to human being."[2(p49)] If the role of the nurse is viewed in such a manner, it is no wonder that nurses wish to move on to better things.

What is nursing? What is the role of the nurse? What is it that makes a nurse a nurse? Is it indeed the functions that we perform? How is it then that the director of nursing service, the administrator of a nursing home, the dean of a college of nursing, the primary care nurse, the operating room nurse, the public health nurse, the psychiatric nurse all claim to be nurses? We perform radically different functions and yet each of us claims the title "nurse." How can it be that those who, in the eyes of the sociologists, have moved beyond nursing still consider themselves nurses? Could it be that rather than evolving out of nursing, these nurses are actualizing new possibilities within nursing?

Could it be that nursing *should not* be defined sociologically, but rather philosophically? Nursing can and should be distinguished by its philosophy of care and *not* by its care functions. Nurses themselves must formulate this philosophy and when they do, they transcend any particular function of nursing only to realize a more developed concept—a concept that embraces and unifies the experience of all nurses rather than denying or denigrating any of that experience.[3]

NURSING—A MORAL ART

The end or purpose of nursing is the welfare of other human beings. This end is not a scientific end, but rather a moral end. That is, it involves the seeking of good and it involves our relationship with other human beings. The science that we learn, the technological skills that we develop are both shaped and designed by that moral end—much as an artist uses a brush. Therefore, nursing is a moral art.[4] The wise and human application of our knowledge and skill is the moral art of nursing. Nursing science serves this art, and this art would not be possible without nursing science. This art is a moral art because it involves other human beings, our relationship with those human beings and the promotion of what we see mutually as "good"—health.

The Concept of Advocacy

Anyone acquainted with the history of nursing is familiar with the various models proposed as models of nursing, such as the nurse as caretaker, the nurse as champion of the sick, the nurse as health educator, the nurse as physician assistant (extender, surrogate, etc.), the nurse as parent surrogate, and the nurse as healer. None of these seems adequate.

Perhaps the philosophical foundation and ideal of nursing is the nurse as *advocate*. The concept of advocacy implied here is not the concept implied in the patients' rights movement nor the legal concept of advocacy, but a far more fundamental advocacy founded upon the simplest and most basic of premises. This concept is not simply one more alternative to be added to the list of past and present concepts of nursing nor does it reject any of them—it embraces all of them. It is not structured rigidly so as to preclude alternatives, rather it involves the basic nature and purpose of the nurse–patient relationship. It is proposed as a very simple foundation upon which the nurse and patient in any given encounter can freely determine the form that relationship is to have, i.e., child and parent, client and counselor, friend and friend, colleague and colleague and so forth through the range of possibilities. This foundation is philosophically prior to any particular relationship and, in fact, enables that relationship to exist.

This proposed ideal of advocacy is based upon our common humanity, our common needs and our common human rights. We are human beings, our patients

---

We are human beings, our patients or clients are human beings, and it is this shared humanity that should form the basis of the relationship between us.

---

or clients are human beings, and it is this commonality that should form the basis of the relationship between us. It often seems that we have permitted traditionalism, elitism and more recently legalism to obscure this most basic of facts.

What It Means to Be a Human Being

To even begin to understand what the human relationship in the professional context means, we have to examine who we are and where we come from. We must approach these questions in the only way we know how, as individuals whose knowing begins with our senses. What we are

examining are human beings, very special kinds of beings who exist in a visible ambience at a determinable point in time and space, beings who know and who know that they know, beings who laugh and cry—and sometimes know why.

Human beings cannot be fragmented. One of our deepest convictions, confirmed by all of our experience, is that each person is a unity.[5] I who think, I who know, I who feel, I who hope, I who fear, I who believe am one! As we grow and mature we come to realize that although we are separate and distinct from all other creatures and the world, we belong to them and with them because we have grown out of the growth of others, learned from their knowledge and benefited from their sufferings. Each person is an integrity, a unity, but a unity that is interrelated and interdependent.

Slowly and painfully, we have come to understand and demand our own dignity. We now know that freedom, respect and integrity are essential to our full development as persons. These concepts have crystallized in what we call human rights.[6] Although it has taken us a bit longer, we now realize that these rights belong to all persons—young and old, black, white, red and yellow; healthy and sick. The progress in this direction has not been smooth, nor is there anything to keep us from backsliding, but progress has been made.[7]

Those concepts we call human rights derive essentially from human needs—*not* human wants, but real, fundamental human needs. Whether the right is physical (such as the right to bodily integrity) or intellectual (such as the right to learn), each is essential to our integrity—our unity—as persons.

HUMAN RIGHTS AND THE NURSE–PATIENT RELATIONSHIP

The relevance of this concept of human rights to the nurse–patient relationship is profound because the patient/client's human needs are magnified by disease. Moreover, the process of the disease itself renders the patient/client far more vulnerable to abuse. Furthermore, the disease process itself may well create new, fundamental needs, needs that must be addressed if the person is to maintain unity-integrity as a unique human being.

Nurses are in a unique position among health professionals to attend the patient/client as a unity because they are able to experience patients as human beings.[3] Not only do nurses attend patients when distress is immediate, but they attend them for sustained periods of time, often providing those intimate details of physical and emotional care that lead to a knowledge of this person as a distinct and unique human being. This knowledge is a precondition for the fundamental type of advocacy referred to here—not legal advocacy, not even health advocacy, but human advocacy.

The only way in which the *unique* human needs of patients or clients can be met is for nurses to attend them as unities. This requires not only an understanding of patients as human beings, but an understanding of each patient as a unique human being. Nurses must be sensitive to individuals and to their reactions to those needs created by illness that threaten the unity or integrity of the person.

Not only must nurses understand the specific physiological damage caused by

disease processes, but they must also understand what illness does to the humanity of the sufferer. The wounds produced by illness stretch far beyond the person's physiological or even psychological limits and penetrate the existential depths of the person's being.[8] These very special wounds create very special needs—needs that must be met if we are to minister to the patient as a human being. These wounds must be addressed if we are to respect the human rights of patients/clients, if we are to accept human advocacy as the foundation of the nurse–patient relationship.

HOW DISEASE DAMAGES OUR HUMANITY

Loss of Independence

One of the very first things that illness does to human beings is to infringe upon their autonomy or independence as people. At the very least, individuals are required to go to another person, to place themselves before this person, to admit that they have a deficiency or a defect and to ask to have it alleviated. In effect, disease makes a petitioner out of an independent individual and threatens the person's self-image. The more personal or more threatening the disclosure is, the more difficult it is for a person to reveal the problem.

Ordinarily, when we meet with a threat we either fight or flee.[9] Yet we cannot flee from ourselves, nor can we fight that within ourselves which we cannot control. This is the ultimate threat, the threat that comes from within, and no matter how hard we try, we cannot have it alleviated without becoming a petitioner. The position of a petitioner is so repugnant to many that they will go to great lengths and take great risks to avoid it. If we are sensitive to this difficulty, the pain it imposes, the humiliation it brings, we can take some steps to alleviate it. So often it seems that health professionals (and nurses are no exception) are so caught up in their own business, their own knowlege and their own self-importance that they fail to consider this first humiliation of the patient or client. We must be willing to unravel the "medical mystique," to become more accessible and to remember that we too are human beings. It is only in doing so that we can begin to heal this first wound to the humanity, to assist individuals to overcome this first obstacle.

Loss of Freedom of Action

The second wound that impinges upon the humanity of the individual is the loss of freedom of action. The human being uses the body to transcend the body itself.[10(p28–29)] That is, unlike animals, we use our bodies for more than the fulfillment of physiological needs and instinctual drives. Human beings are bodily creatures, but they use their bodies to express their hopes, dreams, ideals and values. When we are ill we cannot command our bodies to do what we want them to do and thus in this sense our humanity is wounded, sometimes very seriously.

Insofar as possible we must assist the patient/client to communicate these essential aspects of their humanity. If they cannot do so, we must take steps to discover their value systems and then to respect them. The losses of freedom of action (verbal, locomotive, often intellectual) inflict another wound to the individual's humanity—and sometimes a very serious one!

Interference with Ability to Make Choices

In a third dimension our humanity is damaged by the interference of disease with our ability to make choices—not our right to make choices, but our ability to exercise that right. While there are many factors operant in decision making, it still remains that a decision to be truly valid, must be rational. This is a particularly sensitive area. Often professionals may consider only those decisions that agree with their own to be rational. This is not necessarily the case. However, we must be aware that pain, disability, trauma and drugs all becloud the ability to make choices as does the trauma caused by the loss of wholeness and the loss of ability to act.

Nevertheless, in all circumstances the right to consent rests within the individual. Under certain circumstances we may presume consent; in others we may obtain authorization to act; but the right always remains within the individual. If we are sensitive to this fact, we are far more likely to try to discover and act upon the patient's value system rather than our own or that of significant others. Because this situation has been greatly magnified by our increasing technological power to intervene in an individual's life, the responsibility to discover and respect the patient's value system has assumed vastly increased significance.[11]

Power of Health Care Professionals

A corollary of these factors, and perhaps one of the most devastating attacks on our personhood, is that we are placed in the power of others. Many institutions in society exercise enormous power over us, but these powers have been recognized and surrounded with legal safeguards. It has been widely recognized, for example, that consent obtained under duress is not legally binding.[12] Few things in life are as coercive as the threat of suffering and death (in this instance imposed by illness). Yet what legal advocate, what laws of state, can protect us from these? Thus those persons whom we see as capable of

---

Whether we as health professionals want it or not, whether we like it or not, we exercise enormous power over the people whom we should serve.

---

relieving these threats can and do exercise enormous power over us. Not only do patients, generally speaking, lack the knowledge necessary to define the threat, but they also lack the ability to reduce the threat. Whether we as health professionals want it or not, whether we like it or not, we exercise enormous power over those whom we should serve. How do we use this power? What does this power mean in the light of human advocacy?

RESPONSIBILITIES OF HUMAN ADVOCACY

Information must be provided—at least enough to enable patients/clients to choose among options; but how and when patients/clients are told are at least as significant as what they are told. In the past (and often today), patients were uninformed largely because it was assumed that the health professionals, perhaps in concert with the families, knew what was best for the patients. Usually professionals do know what is best from the technical viewpoint, but it is doubtful that such knowlege extends into the realm of values.

Today, largely because of legal requirements, patients may be subjected to a tyranny of information. More as a hedge against malpractice than out of respect for human rights, patients are fed an enormous, disagreeable and indigestible lump of information-_-and all at one sitting. How much more patients would benefit from small amounts of information provided when they are ready for them and as they ask for them. If nurses and physicians worked collaboratively rather than jealously protecting territorial limits, the patient would greatly benefit. Because nurses have the opportunity to experience the patient as a unique human being and because they spend more time with the patient, nurses can more readily provide information as the patient requests it and when the patient is prepared for it.

Because individuals have been damaged by trauma or disease, and perhaps because they have been placed in the power of others, they have to a large extent *lost their freedom to define for themselves their own image of what it is they should be.* For example, there was a case of a 22-year-old male patient who was diagnosed as having primary cancer of the testes. He was a jockey, a husband and the father of two young sons. There was no evidence of metastasis. He was told of his diagnosis, the need for an orchiectomy and the effect this operation would have on his relationship with his wife. He and his wife discussed the situation and, considering the alternative, decided upon surgery. What he was not told, however, was at least as significant as what he was told. He was not told that he would lose his facial hair, develop breasts and develop a feminine speaking voice. How much did we impinge upon this person's identity? What did we do to his self-image? What image did he present to his sons? To his wife? What kind of comments did he have to endure at the race track? We do not know, but what we do know is that he committed suicide nine months after surgery.

So often by trying to do what we think is right by our value system, we trespass upon the authenticity of the person. Although in many cases our transgressions are not so great, in some cases they are profound. This man's decision might not have been any different if he had known all the facts, but the real question is whether or not the *individual rather than the professional* should make such value decisions. If we decide that a person cannot, how do we reach this conclusion? Can we not, should we not, ought we not assist the patient in decision making AND YET RESPECT THE PATIENT'S DECISION once it is made?

If these wounds are not addressed, and indeed if they are exacerbated, the most devastating of existential wounds develops. Insofar as patients' values are ignored, or replaced with others' values, patients cease to exist as unique human beings. Depersonalization may be partial or complete, but those individuals will die as the persons they were. If the depersonalization is complete, those individuals will not be able to create new values and goals in their life and they will lose a sense of meaning or purpose in their existence.[13] As the philosopher Nietzsche put it, "He who has the why to live can bear with almost any how."[14]

We must—as human advocates—assist patients to find meaning or purpose in their living or in their dying. This can mean whatever the patients want it to mean; it can range from enlisting religious aid to cracking irreverent jokes, from finding a new vocation to adjusting to the old one, from fighting the inevitable to the last breath to complete acceptance of death. Whatever patients define as their goal, it is their meaning and not ours, their values and not ours, and their living or dying and not ours.

Any application of human advocacy is subject to personal and situational interpretation by the practitioner. This is precisely why human advocacy can serve as a foundation upon which any practitioner in any given situation can develop the framework of the nurse–patient relationship according to the unique needs presented by that particular relationship.

According to Garver, violence is not so much a matter of force as it is a matter of violating persons physically, intellectually or psychologically.[15] Certainly not every limitation of a person's autonomy can be seen as an act of violence. To take this position would be to take the moral "punch" out of the notion of psychological violence. For example, one simply cannot equate a regulation limiting how loud patients may tune their television sets with the rendering of patients incompetent in various degrees by withholding information, thus interfering with their rational processes. The concept of psychological violence must be reserved to those cases in which grave or systematic harm is done to the person. The ability to distinguish those cases requires a sensitivity to the human needs created by illness and the unique manifestation of these needs in each patient, NOT IN SERIOUS MATTERS ONLY, but in the daily living experience of patients/clients.

Consider the daily living experience of an institutionalized patient. An individual comes into the patient's room to insert an I.V., and the patient does not even know about the I.V. or why it is being given. Another person comes in to administer a medication that the patient does not even know about or why it is being given. Still another person comes in to catheterize the patient, to administer an enema, to draw blood, to examine every part of the patient's body, to transport the patient here or there for this test or that, and the patient doesn't even know where they are going, what is being done or why it is being done.

Each individual violation may or may not amount to a serious infringement on the patient's autonomy, but collectively they constitute both physical and psychological violence. Note that the effect on the patient is systematic. Confusion, lack of knowledge, lack of explanation, the pervasive assumption that the patient's body belongs to the "professionals" to do with what they will—all lead to reduced possibilities for decision making. Such systematic violation leads to reduced possibilities for making decisions in other,

perhaps critical, areas. Human beings are reduced to objects acted upon, in effect a wholesale reduction of autonomous decision making.[16] Patient and family are thus rapidly socialized into obedience patterns and nonconformity is swiftly punished in both subtle and not so subtle ways.

ESSENCE OF NURSING

Nurses can and do control the environment of the institution, and nurses can institute progressive and humanizing changes if they so desire. Explanations and working together with a patient are not extras that nurses may choose to do, they are the essence of nursing, the essence of

---

Explanations and working together with a patient are not extras that nurses may choose to do; they are the essence of nursing, the essence of the nurse–patient relationship.

---

the nurse–patient relationship. Obviously, in certain critical situations, there is no time for an in-depth discussion of values or even explanations. These circumstances, however, constitute only a minute portion of nurse–patient interactions and should not be used to negate patient rights in the majority of situations.

To claim that nurses can institute progressive change is not to ignore the many organizational and social barriers that nurses face. We can control our own actions. To be sure there are inflexible policies and insensitive orders from physicians, but the professional nurse has a great deal of latitude in the implementation of such policies and orders. Our ethical responsibility is not reduced by the actions of others, but in fact may be magnified by them.[17] Discretion and maturity are necessary components of the truly effective professional.

Nursing and the individual nurse are in very vital positions to help create a climate respectful of the human rights and needs of patients. No other profession and no other professional can exercise as great an influence over the environment of the institution (the environment of the patient) as do the nurse and nursing. If we, as a profession, work together to create an atmosphere that is open to and supportive of the individual's decision making, we may well perform our greatest service to patients/clients and their families.

In many instances nurses are not free to disclose certain information to patients/clients and their families. That is, they are not free unless they are willing to pay the price, a price that may well include loss of employment or even liscensure. This situation is wrong because it violates both the patient's and the nurse's integrity.[18] Moreover, it constitutes a direct infringement of the nurse's right to practice nursing and interferes directly with the nurse–patient relationship.[19] This situation must, can and will be changed.

However, even the existence of such factors does not justify the daily violation of the patient in those matters that nurses do control. It is not an excuse for the psychological violence to which the person is subjected in the daily living experience as an institutionalized patient. The concept of human advocacy transcends even those situational problems created by physicians who knowingly withhold information from patients because it is based on the patient's humanity and the professional's humanity. This is certainly not a complex concept; rather it is so simplistic that it seems almost ludicrous to propose it. All patients—surgical patients, psychiatric patients, medical patients, pediatric patients, dying patients—are still living human beings with all that this implies. If we remember this—and remember too that we are also human beings—the concept of human advocacy is as natural as living and dying.

REFERENCES

1. Schulman, S. "Basic Functional Roles in Nursing: Mother Surrogate and Healer" in Jaco, E., ed. *Patients, Physicians and Illness* (Glencoe, Ill.: The Free Press 1958) p. 528–537.
2. Travelbee, J. *Interpersonal Aspects of Nursing* (Philadelphia: F. A. Davis and Co. 1966).
3. Gadow, S. "Existential Advocacy: Philosophical Foundation for Nursing." Paper presented to the Four State Consortium on Nursing and the Humanities, Phase I Conference, "Nursing and the Humanities: A Public Dialogue," Farmingham, Connecticut, November 11, 1977.
4. Curtin, L. "Nursing Ethics: Theories and Pragmatics." *Nurs Forum* 17:1 (Spring 1978).
5. Chardin, P. de. *The Phenomenon of Man*, Wahl, B., trans. (New York: Harper & Row, Publishers 1959).
6. Dostoevski, F. "Notes from Underground" in *The Short Novels of Dostoevski*, Garnet, C., trans. (New York: Dial Press 1945) p. 149.
7. Dubos, R. *So Human an Animal* (New York: Charles Scribner and Sons 1968) p. 40.
8. Pellegrino, E. "A Humanistic Foundation for Medicine." Paper presented to the Second International Institute of Health Care, Ethics and Human Values, Mount St. Joseph College, Mount St. Joseph, Ohio, July 1976.
9. Gardiner, W. L. *Psychology: A Story of a Search*

(Belmont, Calif.: Brooks/Cole Publishing Co. 1970).

10. Descartes, R. as quoted in Heidegger, M. *Existence and Being* (Chicago: Henry Regnery and Sons 1949) p. 28–29.

11. McCormick, R. Lecture given to the Third International Institute for Health Care, Ethics and Human Values, Mount St. Joseph College, Mount St. Joseph, Ohio, July 1976.

12. Vinogradoff, P. *Collected Papers* vol. 2, ch. 20 (Oxford: Clarendon Press 1928).

13. Frankl, V. E. *Man's Search for Meaning: An Introduction to Logotherapy*, Lasche, I., trans. (New York: Pocket Books 1963) p. 160–163.

14. Nietzsche, F. *The Birth of Tragedy and the Geneology of Morals*, Golffing, F., trans. (Garden City, N. Y.: Doubleday & Co. 1956) p. 299.

15. Garver, N. "What Violence Is." *The Nation* (June 1968) p. 817–822.

16. Curtin, L. "Informed Consent: Information or Exploitation?" *Update on Ethics* 1:4.

17. American Nurses' Association. *Code for Nurses*, articles 1–3 (Kansas City, Mo.: ANA 1976).

18. Curtin, L. "Nursing Ethics: Theories and Pragmatics." *Nurs Forum* 17:1 (Spring 1978), p. 4–11.

19. Curtin, L. "Nursing Practice—A Right and a Duty." *Nurs Ethics* 1:1 (Fall 1978) p. 7–11.

Ethical Choice in Nursing

Paula Sigman R.N., M.S.
Nurse Consultant
Methodist Hospitals of Dallas
Doctoral Candidate
Texas Woman's University
Dallas, Texas

MAKING JUDGMENTS and then deliberately acting upon those judgments is essential to the practice of nursing. Such actions must involve rational thought rather than emotion or intuition; they involve a conscious, cognitive skill necessary to perceive patient needs and provide patient care.[1,2]

Some theorists believe that the most effective, lasting or helpful decisions or judgments are best made with minimal deliberation.[3] Others postulate that the longer a decision takes and the choices are weighed, the greater the efficiency.[4] Most agree, however, that decision making involves talent in reasoning and involves taking risks.[5-7] Others have shown that decisiveness and the commitment to take action defines judgment and allows an individual to engage in the decision-making process.[8,9] In other words, the decision-making process involves deliberative action whereby options and resolutions are considered and the decision is made in terms of one's judgment as to the appropriateness of that choice. In turn, each judgment characteristically involves not only prior judgmental behavior, reaching toward a goal and the "immediacy of the moment," but each judgment also involves an ethical component.[10]

It is a well-acknowledged fact that physicians and professional nurses make decisions daily which affect them, their clients, their profession, the institution in which they practice and, foremost, the quality of care they administer.[1,11,12] Since ethics are generally accepted as a necessary and possibly the most important component of all decisions, recent investigation and literature consequently have shown that responsible decisions made daily by physicians and professional nurses are frequently based upon ethics.[4,10,13-18]

Ethical choice in nursing, as in all areas of health care, is one of the major areas of concern in professional nursing practice. Such issues as accountability, responsibility and even nursing diagnosis have firmly established roots in ethics. "Ethical roots," like the roots of century-old oaks, are neither easily discernible nor easily removed nor destroyed. Instead, they twist and snarl deeper into the surface, often encroaching upon seemingly well-established saplings and neighbors, disturbing even the most solidly built foundations. Attempts to remove them or deny their existence are futile because, regardless of how thorough one is at the attempt, fragments remain and will eventually exert influence.

In order to thoroughly deal with the timely, essential and fundamental issue of ethical choices in nursing, it is important to analyze the definition of responsible

ethical choice, ethical systems upon which ethical choice is based and the validity of teaching ethics to nurses.

DEFINING RESPONSIBLE ETHICAL CHOICE FOR NURSING

Everything is neither right nor wrong. The right or wrong is in the choosing, the keeping, the losing. All paths are light and shadow, and every path is a different thing to each man. The right and the wrong, the good and the evil lie not upon the silent pathway, but in the man that walks it...[19 (p198)]

Decision theory is used today either to focus upon a process concerned with outcomes or to analyze the determinants for individual choice. The second approach not only involves the descriptive or normative rules pertaining to people deciding what is true or what action to take, but also focuses upon the choosing, not the outcome.[20]

Figure 1 presents a model of the types of decisions made and the influences on decisions. Decisions, "resolutions to questions, controversy, disputes or doubt,"[21(p413)] are multidimensional, varying in type from moral to amoral, intelligent to nonreflective, professional to nonprofessional. Furthermore, decisions are influenced by values, beliefs, attitudes, past experiences, morals, knowledge, loves and human philosophy.[9,14,22,23] The last influence, human philosophy, can range anywhere between the two extreme views, between Hobbes and Sartre. Hobbes views society as supreme and law as the pivot point standing between chaos and social functioning.[24] The existentialists, such as Sartre, view the individual as supreme and

FIGURE 1. INFLUENCES ON DECISIONS: A MODEL APPROACH

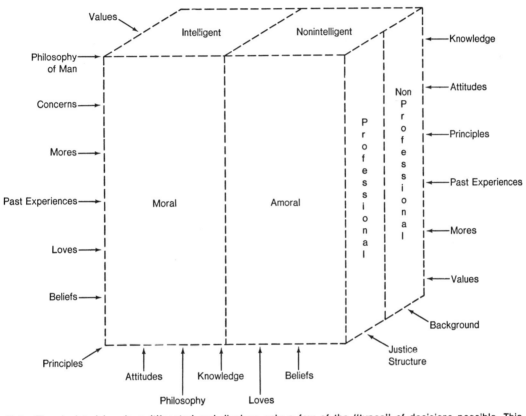

Note: The depicted box is multifaceted and displays only a few of the "types" of decisions possible. This multidimensional approach to decisions also shows how the various types of decisions are not completely distinct—the lines are not solid, accounting for how people might believe themselves to be making one type of decision while in reality they are in another decisional dimension. Numerous biases and other factors (mores, values, beliefs, etc.) are shown to influence all the various types of decisions. Many believe that all types of decisions have ethical components and are influenced, to varying degrees, by the same numerous factors.
Sources:
Boulding, K. E. "The Ethics of Rational Decision." *Management Sci* 12 (1966) p. B161-B169.
Murphy, M. A. and Murphy, J. "Making Ethical Decisions—Systematically" *Nurs '76* (May 1976) p. 13-15.

believe that the individual has the freedom to make of himself what he will.[25]

The middle position between these two extremes, pragmatism, takes both sides into account: A decision is reached that respects both just laws and loves ("loves" are our enduring set of internalized beliefs, attitudes and values).[26,27]

The concept of decision, then, implies change. A decision is a process involving choice, "affected with an ethical interest."[10(p161)] Together with ethical interest, choice and change, goes risk, another essential element in the concept of decision.[11,28]

Yet another element is freedom, the

For professional nurses, decisions are an integral part of daily functioning. Responsible ethical choice based upon responsible ethical behavior involves responsibility, accountability, risk, commitment and justice.

power to determine one's own actions with the absence of or release from ties or obligations that interfere with reasoning. Freedom is closely connected to choice, and controversy exists as to whether there is such a thing as free choice.[26,29] For every act of freedom equal responsibility exists.[30]

For professional nurses, decisions are an integral part of daily fuctioning. Responsible ethical choice based upon responsible ethical behavior involves responsibility, accountability, risk, commitment and justice. These concepts may be defined as follows:

Responsibility requires the capacity for rational, moral decision making.[31] Action itself is not implied but reliability and chargeability are involved; individuals are answerable to something in their own power and control.[32] Responsibility involves accountability.

Accountability signifies action. It is a statement of reasons and consequences whereby nurses may be called upon to account for or explain their actions or position.

Risk is the undertaking of peril, jeopardy or dangerous chance of loss, and is obviously related to accountability.

Commitment means to pledge or align one's self with objects or persons.

Commitment involves self, loyalty and trust.

Justice is the unifying concept or central principle of morality.[34,35] Justice defines morality.[36]

Moral situations can be viewed as conflict-of-interest situations and to resolve these conflicts, principles of justice are then involved. A person's sense of justice is distinctly moral: "One can act morally and question all rules, one may act morally and question the greater good, but one cannot act morally and question the need for justice."[33(p40)]

When speaking of responsible ethical choice in nursing, several assumptions must be made:

1. One has no right to "play it safe."
2. One has no right to benefit self at the expense of others.
3. One must independently formulate a concept of justice.
4. Agreements create obligations which, in turn, create justification.[37]
5. Action is not right if only done through obligation (Plato).
6. One must not allow emotions to dictate to morals or to affect decisions i.e., follow the best reasoning.

The elements of responsible ethical behavior can now be described. Responsible ethical behavior occurs when:

1. A moral principle exists that involves a moral obligation or duty to do or to refrain from doing something that is within the power of the person to do, or is such that the person can do otherwise;
2. Some source of responsibility is

involved as well as a source (hopefully internal) of reward, praise or punishment for responsible action;

3. The cause of the behavior is internal to the individual, i.e., he or she is not compelled by others to act;

4. The behavior itself is not done through ignorance, is respectful of the laws viewed as just by the individual, maintains the integrity and freedom of choice of the "actor" and attempts to do justice to one's loves.[9,14]

In order for responsible ethical choice to occur, certain conditions must exist:

1. The actor is faced with a risky situation, is asked to or is faced with the need to take deliberative action, not merely to respond habitually or mechanically. True choice exists between possible courses of action and the actor places a significantly different value upon each possible action or upon the possible consequences of the action. The actor is accountable for the action taken.

2. A moral principle is involved. A means of achieving ends or goals exists and various alternatives, motives and consequences are available. Also, a commitment is demanded of the actor.

3. The action taken is intelligent, reflective (not blind), free (not forced), just, responsible, consistent with values, consultee-free and it may involve a recipient.[38]

The concept of responsible ethical choice, then, involves a dynamic decision process. While all decisions may involve some sort of ethical component, not all decisions are ethical ones. It is the complete process that not only designates the difference but also moves the individual to continue toward the completion of the process and the making of ethical, responsible choice.

DEFINING ONE'S ETHICAL SYSTEM: THE BASIS OF ETHICAL CHOICE

> Situations do not present themselves with labels attached ... the crux is in the labeling, or the decision ... depends upon how a situation is "seen." [36(p1093)]

In spite of nursing's sometimes precarious position in the health care field, or possibly because of it, professional nurses are daily faced with decisions involving moral and ethical choices. Since the terms *moral* and *ethical* refer to different levels of activity and are not interchangeable, a nurse can be *moral* by acting according to rules of right conduct without being ethical, i.e., to go through the formal reasoning process to decide upon behavior.[40]

This section will (1) show the necessity for and the development of each individual professional nurse's ethical system, for without the use of a formal, rational ethical system, decisions made by the nurse are not ethical although they may be moral, and (2) since nurses are often called upon not only to make an ethical decision but to explain that decision, knowing the ethical theories and being able to articulate them, the professional nurse gives substance and support to the decision and is afforded increased security in his or her knowledge of the reason behind the action.

As stated earlier, the terms *moral* and *ethical* are not interchangeable. Ethics is considered one of the three branches of philosophy; the other two are metaphysics, dealing with theories of reality; and epistemology, which distinguishes between knowledge and belief. Ethics deals with the values of human life in a coherent, systematic and logical manner. It is concerned with the type of conduct that is judged as right or wrong or good or bad. In other words, ethics deals with practical problems that arise from human conduct when an individual is faced with a choice between alternative values. Individuals must decide among several possible alternatives what to do in a given situation; they must decide upon the best action to take in spite of conflicting choices that confront them.

Every question of ethics weighs the values involved in problems of choice. An ethical problem, with its two essential ingredients, *choice* and the *valuing* of actions and their consequences, is considered both general, since it involves a vast assortment of moral acts, and theoretical, because it calls upon and leads to ethical theories. Ethics, then, systematically seeks a critical grasp of the principles and standards that help in making morally right choices.

Two basic assumptions are inherent in understanding ethical choice: (1) "Each day man makes innumerable decisions and some are involved with truly moral problems;"[9(p47)] and (2) "An individual can avoid a moral issue that plagues and perplexes others but no competent human being can completely escape the necessity of making responsible ethical decisions."[41(p14)]

Accordingly, the moral sphere includes only acts that are not trivial, that affect both an agent and others and that are matters of conscience. In turn, moral problems are specific (not general), employ the word *ever* and arise from practical decisions with answers readily applicable to future practice.[41] For example, is the taking of human life ever justifiable?

Therefore, working through a moral problem causes normative questions to arise that reaffirm a norm by which both the "rightness" and "wrongness" of an act and the values attached to objects of the act can be judged. For instance, from the moral problem "Is the taking of a human life ever justifiable?" naturally comes the normative question "What makes an act right or wrong?" That question is answered by the theory of obligation to which one subscribes. A moral problem such as "Is LSD of value to man?" leads to the theoretical normative question "What is intrinsically good?" That question is born of one's accepted theory of value.

By wedding theory of obligation and theory of value, an ethical system is

---

By wedding theory of obligation and theory of value, an ethical system is formed. The task is to combine the two into a system of moral philosophy that will adequately answer daily moral questions.

---

formed. In other words, a theory of value is necessary to complete a theory of obligation. The task is to combine the two into a system of moral philosophy that will adequately answer daily moral questions.

What, then, are the theories of obligation and value that together form an ethical system?

Theories of Obligation

Theories of obligation, i.e., "What makes an act right or wrong?," define the right- or wrong-making characteristics of an act as grounds of obligation. Eight theories of obligation are generally accepted to describe the possible approaches in determining what makes an act right or wrong.

The *one-characteristic-of-an-act* theory of obligation states that one and only one feature, regardless of the complexities surrounding the problem, makes an act right or wrong. For instance, to kill is wrong regardless of whether the killer is an adult or a child, the aggressor or the attacked, whether the act is done spontaneously or is premeditated. The single feature says that to take a human life, no matter what the circumstances, is still wrong by virtue of its intrinsic nature.[42]

The major argument against this approach is that the theory oversimplifies morality when conflicting obligations exist. For example, a nurse has contracted with an outside agency to work with an evening outpatient group of depressed individuals. One day an emergency arises on an acute care unit where she is a clinical specialist; she chooses to stay and deal with the emergency. She never arrives at the group session across town and is unable to notify anyone of the problem. Accordingly, to account for the complexity of moral choices evident in this example, another theory must be considered.

The *one-or-more-characteristics-of-an-act* theory of obligation states that what makes an act right or wrong is intrinsic to the nature of the action itself, and is not external to it. This approach, however, denies that only one characteristic feature of obligation exists. According to this theory, the agent must weigh the key features of the problem and do what has the greatest obligation of rightness; he or she must consider if the right outweighs the wrong.[43] For instance, consider again the dilemma facing the clinical specialist with conflicting obligations: which action—to stay for the obvious crisis or to leave and avert a potential crisis with the outpatient group—has the greatest obligation of rightness? Which right-making characteristics outweigh the wrong-making ones?

The *agent's welfare* is a third theory of obligation. Also known as *ethical egoism,* this theory postulates that right or wrong is determined by the agent's welfare and the impact the action or lack of action will have on his or her welfare. The major underlying premise is that the act that is most advantageous and beneficial to the agent is the right one.[26] For instance, is one obligated to always tell the truth? Is it right to tell a "little white lie" to save embarrassment when no one will know the difference or be hurt by it? Is the physician who pockets charges without recording and reporting them to the Internal Revenue Service rightfully obligated to report and record this additional income?

Act utilitarianism is the theory of obligation that states that the rightness or wrongness of an act depends upon the degree to which it is harmful or useful. For instance, telling the truth is right because it is useful, and falsehoods are wrong because of their harmful effects.

The October issue of *Nursing '74* reported on the honesty of nurses. Based on 11,681 replies, 70% of the nurses admitted to regularly taking hospital supplies ranging from aspirin and antacid to linens and surgical supplies; economic considerations alone can speak to the harmful effects of this practice.

Rule utilitarianism states that an act is right or wrong depending upon whether it conforms to or violates a moral rule. In turn, a moral rule is justified or unjustified depending on its utility or desirability, thus avoiding problems with act utilitarianism. For example, it is wrong to not tell the truth *except* to save a life or spare someone's feelings.[44(p410)]

Universalizability states that what makes an act right is the ability to universalize its maxim; a wrong act is not universalizable.[45] For example, nothing is gained by cheating since we do not want everyone to cheat and it is morally wrong to make one's self an exception; therefore, since we *cannot* universalize and say cheating should be done by everyone, cheating is wrong. Universalizability, then, distinguishes right from wrong. The theory's strength seems to lie in the way in which it "captures the essence of morality," for to act morally means to act on principle.[41]

Obligation by *mores* and the *dictates of the law of God*, are also theoretical approaches to the rightness or wrongness of an act. Both theories strongly address the bindingness of obligation. Anthropologists such as William Sumner maintain that mores make an act right or wrong; man should abide by customs that are socially sanctioned, or mores. For example, if our culture took the maxim "an eye for an eye..." literally, we would cut off our hands because we stole bread to feed our family.

The theory of *the law of God* provides for man a standard of right and wrong above society and temporal concerns. According to this theory, what determines an act to be right or wrong does not lie in the nature of the act itself, an act is right or wrong because God so says through the Bible, His representatives on earth, etc. Strong criticism is directed to this theory of obligation, since the determination of right or wrong is seen by some to be closely related to the nature of the act itself.

It is not enough to act solely upon a theory of obligation; concerns about value easily arise when considering obligation. Every ethical problem faced by an individual is a combination of *choice* between what "should" or "ought to" be done (theory of obligation) and *judgment* about the value of the chosen action (theory of value).

Theories of Value

Theories of value question what makes an act morally good or evil. Numerous approaches to theories of value exist and several will be highlighted here. These theories each point to the one "thing" of value upon which determination of good and evil can be made.

Love, according to many moralists, makes an act virtuous. What determines the moral value of an act is not conformity to external laws of either God or society, but the spirit in which it is done. If all human life becomes the object of agape love (the selfless concern for well-being of others), then actions, dictated by the love, will be virtuous.

Conscientiousness, according to Kant, is the sense of duty which motivates an individual to act. Love, on the other hand, is seen as an unreliable motive because it can lead the moral agent to act in violation of duty. Duty to family, to self, to job, etc., are all motivators to act virtuously—to do good and refrain from evil.

Both *actual value of consequences* and *intended consequences* are theories of value addressed by and to moralists, philosophers and theologians. Righteousness, power, pleasure, motives etc. can be used to explain what it is that makes a thing desirable or undesirable, good or bad. Since ethics is a rational process concerned with determining the best course of action in the face of choices which conflict, part of this rational process is an evaluation of the rules and principles that guide the individual's conduct, actions and decisions. Part of this evaluation is for the individual to answer "What is intrinsically good?" and "What makes an act good as opposed to evil?" In addition, some awareness of what makes an act right or wrong must be arrived at.

In the end, every ethical problem faced by an individual is tied to both the problem of *choice* between what "should" or "ought" to be done (theory of obligation) and *judgment* about the action chosen, usually expressed as "good," "bad," "admirable," etc. (theory of value). The wedding of the two, then, constitutes not only the core of normative ethics but provides the framework for understanding the ethical system used to make responsible ethical choices.

CAN AND SHOULD RESPONSIBLE ETHICAL BEHAVIOR BE TAUGHT TO PROFESSIONAL NURSES?

> Each of us should lay aside all other learning, to study how . . . to distinguish the good life from the evil.[46(p310)]
>
> Ethical judgments are neither true or false, they are not the sort of things that can be known, learned or doubted.[41(p291)]

Baccalaureate nursing educators profess to educate students in decision making as beginning practitioners in the nursing profession.[47,48] Throughout such nursing curricula emphasis is placed upon the decision-making process and the exercise of concise and pertinent nursing judgments.[49-51] However, from both a random hand survey of accredited baccalaureate nursing curricula in the United States in February 1978 and the results of a recent study by the Hastings Center in August 1977, one major component of this decision-making process, ethics, appears to be ignored, only slightly touched upon, or haphazardly included within the curriculum. If included, education in ethics appears limited to a few lectures on the ethical components of decision making, usually presented within the last year of the baccalaureate nursing program.

Few of the accredited colleges or universities in the United States that offer degrees in nursing require specific courses in ethics, ethical choice and the like. Those that do may do so because of pressures from the overall university with its own requirements, as part of a course or courses in the legality of nursing practice or nursing research, or because there is some acknowledgement of the importance of ethical concerns in all nursing judg-ments.[15,52] On the other hand, those that do not include required courses in ethics in their curricula may do so from igno-rance, from fear or inability to make or to introduce major changes in their pro-grams, or because they subscribe to the theory that moral development and subse-quential ethical behavior has its roots early in the developmental process where values are given base and structure and so it is useless to include these courses in a college curriculum.

If it is true that values, beliefs and ideals are formed early in life and therefore are unaffected by courses or even role models, courses in ethics might, at best, only broaden the knowledge base of the nurse and stimulate some questions and insights into existing behaviors, or, at least, provide a few additional credits toward gradua-tion.

Much recent literature has concerned itself with modern American society, its decreasing morality and prolonged adoles-cence.[53-55] If emotional development is prolonged and the stages are not as evident or diagrammatic as proposed by major developmental theorists, perhaps the same can be said of the moral devel-opment of the individual in modern Amer-ican society. Perhaps many individuals either do not attain the final stages of moral development where change or alter-ation is next to impossible and are in effect arrested in their moral development.[34,56] If this is so, could not the individual be either educated or internally (morally) affected by formal education in ethics during baccalaureate nursing education?

If the end products of a baccalaureate nursing program are novice professionals

If the end products of a baccalau-reate nursing program are novice professionals who are capable of ex-ercising reasonable clinical and pro-fessional judgments and who are not limited to common, recurrent prob-lems, are they not decision makers?

who are capable of exercising reasonable clinical and professional judgments and are not limited to common, recurrent problems as are students in the associate degree program, are they not decision makers? And, as decision makers, are not graduating baccalaureate nurses expected not only to display but to use leadership qualities?

Recent professional literature shows that professional schools of medicine, dentis-try, law, etc., are increasingly including courses in ethics. Professional nursing should not imitate other professional schools, for nursing is itself unique and can stand alone. But baccalaureate nursing education, in its premise that it turns out leaders in the field, change agents and decision makers, should consider all aspects of the decision-making process, including ethics.

Some questions must be asked: (1) Is it possible to effect ethical changes in adults? (2) Can and should formal courses in ethics be included in baccalaureate nursing education? (3) If so, when within the baccalaureate nursing education pro-gram should these courses begin, and who should teach them?

While it is rare that any student who enters college today does not have some preliminary, elementary exposure to the scientific method and basic ethical considerations in research and inquiry, ethics, as an essential element in this process, appears to be missing.[18,57] Fundamental ethical behavior and thought has also, to date, been neglected. However, several federally funded programs have begun during the last five years in an attempt to begin to teach the child ethics and ethical behavior early in formal education. Curricula in secondary education and beyond has either included ongoing practical ethics courses or, at least, planned for future courses. Professional schools are also gradually including more and more seminars in ethics as well as practical ethics courses.[58-61]

Professional nursing education, i.e., baccalaureate nursing education, has been slow to follow the example set by other professional schools and suggestions made by some of nursing's own leaders.[62,63] While the American Nursing Association (ANA), in 1977–78, has listed ethics as a priority in terms of research, little evidence of additional courses in ethics exists.[18,57,64]

In the United States, as reported by Virginia Ohlson to the International Council of Nurses, 280 accredited basic nursing education programs in colleges and universities grant the baccalaureate degree. The Goldman Study in 1923, the Brown Report in 1948 and the Bridgman Report in 1953 each identified the need to place nursing education in colleges and universities rather than keep it within hospitals. In 1966, the ANA's "Position Paper on Nursing Education" declared that the nurse should be educated in colleges and universities and, beginning in 1972, a noticeable trend toward preference for baccalaureate education for nurses has been noted. Since the National League for Nursing (NLN) and ANA standards for baccalaureate nursing education emphasize the education of students as decision makers, all aspects of the decision-making process should be included in the curricula. Ethics is one part, and not a small part, of the decision-making process, and thereby, should be included in baccalaureate nursing curricula.[10,13,60]

However, in the United States no national nursing curriculum requirements exist, and the requirements that do exist are the responsibility of each individual state through its state board of nursing. As an academic discipline, nursing is obliged to preserve liberal education and provide, at the least, background basics in the arts and philosophy.[49,63] Some specific trends are evident in baccalaureate curricula and these include provision for more learning experiences so that future professional nurses can make more competent, definitive judgments based upon their increased responsibility in the management of patient care.

Even as early as 1923 Goldman suggested that ethics and the teaching of practical ethics courses be part of baccalaureate nursing education and recent goal overviews also suggest ethical development as a measureable objective for baccalaureate nursing education. But the same questions reoccur: (1) To what extent should practical and theoretical ethics courses be required in baccalaureate nursing curricula? and, (2) If so offered, can such courses have any lasting effect on baccalaureate students whose values, beliefs and ethics may have been solidified early in their development?

Vital to the survival of one's ideals,

values, beliefs and ethics is culture.[65-67] While morality embraced by a culture must be both "flexible and stable enough to adequately respond to the challenges of the time," it must include discipline in its socialization.[66(p97),68] In our modern American society this socialization has become increasingly dependent upon curricula in formal education establishments. Formal education now appears to be the primary means of socialization in our society and is viewed, consequently, as a moral task concerned with the development of moral conciousness and moral character.[60,69,70]

Others have postulated and documented that moral development is sequential, observable and eventual.[34,56] Philip Rieff has stated, "Morality is largely developmental in character ... (and) grows and evolves as does the body. Each stage of moral growth demands its own distinct education, as does the body, and is best nurtured by different foods and regimens during its various stages."[71(p11)]

In other words, morality evolves at different stages with education helping to foster the behavior that is appropriate to each stage. According to Max Weber, the "fostering of moral consciousness in the educational system is as much an art as a science and finds its best setting in the confines of the university."[72] Parsons maintains that the school not only universalizes the socialization pattern but helps children to internalize a level of social values and norms a step higher than those they can learn from the family.[66] Other writers contend that while role requirements and attitudes are internalized fairly early in life, internalization comes later. Fischer points to the dichotomy in modern schools whereby values and expectations are inconsistent in the education of children from the first grade on.[73]

The teaching of values, beliefs and ethics has often been regarded as outside the scope of education for several reasons. First, the idea prevails that values and ethics belong to the innate aspects of the personality that are "impervious to change by educational method."[75(p17)] Secondly, the techniques of teaching and curriculum development have proven to be too crude to provide adequate methodology for teaching values and ethics and evaluating the impact of such teaching methods. However, values and ethics are implicit not only in the functioning of a culture but in institutional dynamics and the forms of education. The education of values and ethics is all pervasive and for the most part unconscious. The task of education is to "make this process conscious, rationally defensible, and as far as the role of curriculum is concerned, more effective."[68(p48)]

In the classical sense, according to Durkheim, to know means to know the reason for, to understand something in terms of its causes.[75] Therefore, it is by explanation, questioning and critical analysis of moral principles that moral knowledge is internalized and effectively actualized as *ethical behavior*. In addition, an individual must be far enough along in intellectual development to be able to synthesize, internalize and effectively use this knowledge through rational processes.

Significance: A Possible Answer

Questions such as "when does moral education occur?" and concerns about whether or not ethics and values courses taught in higher education curricula can have an impact on adult student behavior, are of contemporary significance, especially for the student professional. The underlying theme, however, is far from a contemporary concern; centuries ago a student of Socrates asked, "Can you tell me whether virtue is acquired by teaching or by practice; or if neither by teaching or practice, then whether it comes to man by nature, or in what other way."[76(p799)]

Socrates responded that far from knowing the answer to the question posed, "I'm not even sure of what virtue (morality) is. . . . Is any man?" As would be expected, this topic continues to raise interesting questions for contemporary professional nursing education but remains a question which is still inconclusive in its answer.

In order, then, to include "ethical teaching" in a curriculum, identifiable need must be evident and the following assumptions must be made:

1. It is possible to influence and develop responsible ethical behavior through courses offered in baccalaureate programs and beyond.

2. Professional nurses are increasingly aware of the ethical dimensions of their work and recognize ethics as at least a major influencing factor if not an essential component of the decision-making process.

3. Ethics courses can, at least, foster greater ethical consciousness by teaching nurses both to think critically about situations presented and actions taken, and to recognize some common link in ethical dilemmas.

4. And, as Aristotle has stated in *Nichomachean Ethics*, "Experience *can* promote ethical intelligence."[39(p1094)]

Once the preceding assumptions have been accepted, curriculum development of courses in ethics can begin. Those planning such courses must recognize for what and to whom a professional nurse can be ethically responsible. In other words, the professional nurse's role, limitations within that role and unique areas of ethical responsibility and possible ethical dilemmas must be identified. *Nursing ethics is different from biomedical ethics, not in process but in substance.* Therefore, curricula

Curricula for ethics programs for nursing should reflect the nature of ethical dilemmas faced by nurses and, ideally, should be developed for clinical settings as well as formal class discussion.

should reflect the nature of ethical dilemmas faced by nurses (as opposed to other disciplines) and, ideally, should be developed for clinical settings as well as formal class discussion (of principles, case histories, etc.).

Each curricula must both address and concretely answer the problems of (1) who will teach courses in ethics; (2) how much priority must be given to development of such courses; (3) how can ethics courses become a valued part of the curriculum; and (4) in what way and to what extent can development of an integrated ethics program occur within the entire curriculum? These are fundamental questions to answer in order for ethics to be included in a curriculum. They naturally lead to the less philosophical and more concrete, equally difficult questions concerning format, specific content, scheduling, crediting and evaluating "performance."

Most educators are aware that basic moral and ethical values are acquired by a combination of deliberate teaching and subtle interaction, role modeling and trial-and-error experience. Critical analysis of moral behavior (ethics) is a process that can be influenced beyond the time when basic foundations are set; the ethical process can be taught later in life either to make up for deficiencies in basic moral

education or to bring into focus ethical guidelines by which true critical analysis can result.

The need exists for decision makers in nursing to develop responsible ethical behavior as part of their natural decision-making repertoire. Ethical dilemmas are a daily reality facing professional nurses. Therefore, active movement toward teaching ethics in professional nursing curricula is a key step toward helping future practitioners deal with ethical problems.

REFERENCES

1. Hansen, A. C. and Thomas, D. B. "A Conceptualization of Decision-Making." *Nurs Res* 17:5 (September/October 1968) p. 436–443.
2. Hammond, K. R. et al. "Clinical Inference in Nursing: Use of Information-Seeking Strategies by Nurses." *Nurs Res* 15:4 (Fall 1966) p. 330–336.
3. Atthowe, J. M. "Interpersonal Decision Making: The Resolution of Dyadic Conflict." *J Abn & Soc Psych* 62:12 (1961) p. 114–119.
4. Raz, J. "Reasons for Action, Decisions, and Norms." *Mind* 84:336 (October 1975) p. 481–499.
5. Sarbin, T. R. et al *Clinical Inferences and Cognitive Theory* (New York: Holt, Rinehart and Winston 1960).
6. Kaplin, M. F. and Schwartz, S. *Human Judgment and Decision Processes* (New York: Academic Press 1975).
7. Plax, T. G. and Rosenfeld, L. B. "Correlates of Risky Decision-Making." *J Personal Assess* 40:4 (1976) p. 413–418.
8. Weissman, M. S. "Decisiveness and Psychological Adjustment." *J Psychol Assess* 40:4 (1976) p. 403–412.
9. Stevens, E. *Making Moral Decisions* (New York: Paulist Press 1969).
10. Boulding, K. E. "The Ethics of Rational Decision." *Management Sci* 12 (1966) p. B161–B169.
11. Callahan, D. and Engelhardt, H. T. *Science, Ethics and Medicine* vol. 1 (New York: The Institute of Society, Ethics and the Life Sciences 1976).
12. Doona, M. E. "The Judgement Process in Nursing." *Nurs Outlook* (June 1976) p. 21–24.
13. Doob, L. W. *Pathways to People* (New Haven, Conn.: Yale University Press 1975).
14. Kattsoff, L. O. *Making Moral Decisions: An Existential Analysis* (The Hague: Martinue Hijhoff 1965).
15. Fishburn, P. *Decisions and Value Theory* (New York: John Wiley and Sons 1964).
16. Rabb, J. D. "Implications of Moral and Ethical Issues of Nurses." *Nurs Forum* 15:2 (1976) p. 169–180.
17. Brody, H. *Ethical Decisions* (Boston: Little, Brown and Co. 1976).
18. Steinfels, M. O. "Ethics, Education and Nursing Practice." *Hastings Center Rep* 7:4 (August 1977) p. 20–21.
19. Rogers, G. *Nakoa: Blackfoot Philosophy* (New York: Warner Books 1972).
20. Scheibe, K. *Beliefs and Values* (New York: Holt, Rinehart and Winston 1970).
21. Plax, T. G. and Rosenfeld, L. B. "Correlates of Risky Decision-Making." *J Personal Assess* 40:4 (1976) p. 413–418.
22. Jeffrey, R. C. *The Logic of Decision* (New York: McGraw-Hill Book Co. 1965).
23. Potter, V. R. *Bioethics: Bridge to the Future* (Englewood Cliffs, N.J.: Prentice-Hall 1971).
24. Hobbes, T. *Leviathan* (London: Molesworth Press 1841 original, 1955 reprint).
25. Sartre, J. P. *Existentialism*. Frechtman, B., trans. (New York: Philosophical Library 1947).
26. Frankena, W. K. and Granrose, J. T. *Introductory Readings In Ethics* (Englewood Cliffs, N.J.: Prentice-Hall 1974).
27. Dewey, J. *Human Nature and Conduct* (New York:

Holt, Rinehart and Winston 1922 original, 1976 reprint).

28. Callahan, D. *Ethical Responsibility in Science in the Face of Uncertain Consequences* (New York: Institute of Society, Ethics and the Life Sciences June 1972) p. 1–13.

29. Lemmon, J. "Moral Dilemmas." *Philosoph Rev* LXXI (1962) p. 110–115.

30. Kierkegaard, S. *Either/Or*. Swenson, D. F., trans. (Princeton, N.J.: University Press 1959).

31. Russell, B. *An Outline of Philosophy* (New York: New American Library 1960).

32. Allen, M. "Ethics of Nursing Practice." *Canad Nurse* (February 1974) p. 22–24.

33. Lickona, T. *Moral Development and Behavior: Theory, Research and Social Issues* (New York: Holt, Rinehart and Winston 1976) p. 40.

34. Kohlberg, L. "Development of Moral Character and Moral Ideology" in Hoffman and Hoffman, eds. *Review of Child Development Research* (New York: Russell Sage 1964).

35. Kohlberg, L. and Turiel, E. *Recent Research in Moral Development* (New York: Holt, Rinehart and Winston 1971).

36. Rawls, J. "Two Concepts of Rules." *Philosoph Rev* IXIV (1955).

37. Bach, K. "When To Ask, 'What if everyone did that?'" *Philosoph and Phenomenol Res* 37:4 (June 1977) p. 464–499.

38. Lamont, W. C. *The Principles of Moral Judgment* (Oxford: Clarenden Press 1946).

39. Aristotle. *Nichomachean Ethics* Ross, W. D., trans. (Oxford: Clarenden Press 1915).

40. Aiken, H. *Reason in Conduct: New Bearing in Moral Philosophy* (New York: Knox Publishers 1962) p. 42.

41. Wellman, C. *Moral and Ethics* (Glenview, Ill.: Scott, Foresman and Co. 1975).

42. Silby-Bigge, L. A., ed. *The British Moralists* (New York: Dover Publications 1965).

43. Ross, W. D. "What Makes Right Acts Right?" *The Right and The Good* (Oxford: Clarenden Press 1930) p. 16–47.

44. Jones, W. T. et al. *Approaches to Ethics* (New York: McGraw-Hill Book Co. 1969).

45. Margolis, J., ed. *Contemporary Ethical Theory: A Book of Readings* (New York: Random House 1966).

46. Plato. *The Republic* Lindsay, A. D., trans. (London: J. M. Bent & Sons Ltd. 1935).

47. National League for Nursing. *Criteria for the Appraisal of Baccalaureate and Higher Degree Programs in Nursing* (New York: Council of Baccalaureate and Higher Degree Programs 1976).

48. American Nurses' Association. *Guidelines for Nurs-*

ing Baccalaureate Programs (Kansas City, Mo.: ANA 1975).

49. Guinee, K. K. *The Aims and Methods of Nursing Education* (New York: MacMillan, Inc. 1966).

50. National League for Nursing. *State-Approved Schools of Nursing - R.N., 1977* (New York: NLN Publication 1977).

51. Yera, H. et al. *Nursing Leadership: Theory and Process*. (New York: Appleton-Century-Crofts 1976).

52. Paterson, J. G. and Zderad, L. *Humanistic Nursing* (New York: John Wiley & Sons 1976).

53. Titus, H. and Keeton, M. *Ethics for Today* (New York: D. Van Nostrand 1973).

54. Bok, S. *Lying: Moral Choice in Public and Private Life* (New York: Pantheon Press 1978).

55. Vidal, G. *Kalki* (New York: Random House 1978).

56. Piaget, J. *The Moral Judgment of the Child* (Glencoe, Ill.: Free Press 1948).

57. Aroskar, M. A. "Ethics in the Nursing Curriculum." *Nurs Outlook* 25:4 (April 1977) p. 260–264.

58. Brody, H. "Teaching Medical Ethics—Future Challenges." *J Am Med Assoc* 29:2 (July 8, 1974) p. 177–179.

59. Trow, M. "Higher Education and Moral Development." *The AAUP Bulletin* (Spring 1976) p. 25.

60. Beck, C. M. et al, eds. *Moral Education: Interdisciplinary Approach* (New York: Newman Press 1976).

61. Weisensee, M. G. "The Student's Need for and Right to a 'Holistic' Education." *International Council of University Teachers* (Summer 1977) p. 137–142.

62. Rogers, M. E. *Educational Revolution in Nursing* (New York: MacMillan, Inc. 1961).

63. Machan, L. "The Obligation of Nursing as an Academic Discipline to Preserve Liberal Education." *Nurs Forum* XVI:2 (1977) p. 196–199.

64. Aroskar, M. A. and Veatch, R. "Ethics Teaching in Nursing Schools." *Hastings Center Rep* VII:4 (August 1977) p. 23–27.

65. Mead, M. "The Impact Of Culture on Personality Development in the U.S." *Understand the Child* XX (January 1951) p. 18–26.

66. Parsons, T. "The School Class as a Social System: Some of its Functions in American Society." *Harv Educ Rev* XXIX (Fall 1959) p. 16–24.

67. Kreyche, G. F. and Kopan, A. T. "Value Education and the Private College." *Philosoph Res and Anal* VI:5 (Winter 1976) p. 2–5.

68. Taba, H. *Curriculum Development: Theory and Practice* (New York: Harcourt, Brace and World 1962).

69. Buber, M. "The Education of Character" in *Man and Man* (New York: MacMillan, Inc. 1965).

70. Meyer, J. R., ed. *Reflections on Values Education* (Ontario: Welfred Laurier University Press 1976).

71. Rieff, P. *Moral Choices in Contemporary Society* (Palo Alto, Calif.: Delmar Publications 1977).

72. Weber, M. *The Methodology of the Social Sciences* (Glencoe, Ill.: Free Press 1949).

73. Fischer, M. S. "Children in the World Today" in Linton, R. et al., eds. *Culture and Personality* (Washington, D.C.: American Council on Education 1963).

74. Linton, R. et al. *Culture and Personality* (Washington, D.C.: American Council on Education 1963).

75. Durkheim, E. *Moral Education* (New York: Free Press 1961).

76. Socrates quoted from *Dialogues of Plato* 3rd ed. (Oxford: Oxford University Press, reprint 1932).

Moral Development: A Differential Evaluation of Dominant Models

Anna Omery, MS
Doctoral Candidate
Boston University
School of Nursing
Boston, Massachusetts
Assistant Professor
University of Lowell
Department of Nursing
Lowell, Massachusetts

Can you tell me, Socrates, whether virtue is acquired by teaching or practice; or if neither by teaching or practice, then whether it comes to man by nature or in what other way?[1]

SINCE THE ERA OF Florence Nightingale, the nursing profession has been concerned that its individual members be virtuous. It has only been since the mid-1970s, however, that nursing has begun to actively investigate the process by which these virtues are to be acquired. During the intervening time period, the profession's concern with moral development was manifested primarily in stressing in both the student and the practicing professional the virtues of loyalty, duty, subservience, and blind obedience to authority.

In my estimation, obedience is the first law and the very cornerstone of good nursing. The first and most helpful criticism I ever received from a doctor was when he told me that I was supposed to be simply an intelligent machine for the purpose of carrying out his orders.[2(p394)]

This view of the nurse and of the virtues to be emphasized in the professional role resulted in many early texts on nursing ethics being concerned primarily with "how tos" and "when tos," such as how to baptize the baby and when to call the clergy or physician.

Evolving changes in society and the profession of nursing have made the blind use of such virtues dysfunctional. Current nursing practice mandates a morally responsible professional who is an advocate for the client and a guardian of client rights. Issues in morality have become an integral part of the relationships between nurses and their colleagues and clients. Nurses are frequently placed in situations in which independent moral judgments are required. They must be able to engage in moral reasoning based on moral values and principles that are separate from authority.[3]

Concurrent with this increasing awareness and acceptance of moral responsibility has been a growing concern within the profession that the process of moral development be identified so that the evolution of moral reasoning can be facilitated in both nurses and the clients they service. It is to accommodate this process of facilitation that this evaluation of the dominant models of moral development has been formulated. It seems cogent to begin by delineating moral development.

MORAL DEVELOPMENT

Gilligan[4] has formalized moral development as the "expanding conception of the social world as it is reflected in the understanding and resolution of the inevitable conflicts that arise between self and oth-

ers."[4(p483)] Inherent in this definition is the concept of moral development as a process of learning to resolve social conflict. However, are all social conflicts moral conflicts? If there is disagreement between colleagues about the length they should cut their hair, are they in a moral dilemma? One thinks not; rather, the dilemma seems to be an aesthetic one.

Others have been identified as viewing moral development as the process of internalizing culturally given external rules.[5] Such a definition would view morality as that which is culturally mandated. Under such a definition, the extermination of whole ethnic groups and intellectual populations under the Nazi regime during World War II could conceivably be considered moral. Yet, those actions were and are abhorrently immoral. The perceived difficulty that emerges is not in recognizing that moral development is a process but rather in discovering what is meant by moral.

Shiveder, Turiel, and Much[6] have identified six criteria by which prescriptions may be classified as moral. Prescriptions are moral when they are

1. obligatory—when duties are involved that do not depend on what one wants to do;
2. generalizable—what is right or wrong for one is right or wrong for all in a similar situation; and
3. important—what is moral has precedence.

If obligation is divided into component parts, being moral is

4. impersonal—right or wrong, whether people recognize it as such;
5. unalterable—what is right or wrong does not depend on consensus; and

6. ahistoric—though its recognition may be historic, there is no point in time at which the validity of what is right or wrong changes.

Although he does not delineate criteria, Thiroux[7] has proposed that to be moral is to be ethical; ie, they are synonomous. There are others, however, who disagree. Kudzma[8] sees being moral as determining the right or wrong of a given situation, whereas ethics is used to describe the general nature of morals and moral choice. Thompson and Thompson[9] view morals as the oughts and shoulds of society, whereas they view ethics as the principles, the whys, behind the moral code. Similarly, Beauchamp and Childress[10] define moral rules as actions of a certain kind that ought or ought not to be done because they are right or wrong, whereas they consider ethical principles to be more general and fundamental than the moral rules serving as their foundation. Being moral for these authors appears to reside in the identification of certain action guides, such as "Thou shalt not kill," which are based on such ethical principles as justice, utility, or equality.

In addition, Chazan[11] has identified four criteria that must be present in a given situation for the moral action guides to be appropriately applied.

1. The individual must be faced with a human confrontation or conflict of needs.
2. The decision to be made must be guided by universal principles.
3. The decision must be freely and consciously chosen.
4. The choice is affected by feelings brought by the individual and relating to the particular context of the situation, eg, the time of the day or the appearance of the client.

Using the criteria developed in the preceding discussions, it becomes possible to elucidate moral development as the process of internalizing suggestions or action guides that are obligatory (impersonal, unalterable, or ahistoric), generalizable, and important. These action guides are, furthermore, based on ethical principles such as justice or utility and are used in a specific type of situation.

Models of moral development

Three theories of the personality have been primarily responsible for the emergent operationalization of prevailing models of moral development. These three theories of personality and their respective models of moral development are psychoanalytic, cognitive development, and social learning theory.

Psychoanalytic models

Classic psychoanalytic theory divides the human personality into three structures, the id, the ego, and the superego. Moral development is the result of the development of the last of the structures, the superego. This development results from the resolution of the Oedipus complex and castration anxiety. Since the process is different in males and females, the end product, the superego, is different.[12-17]

For both males and females, the mother's nurturing and close intimacy during infancy result in her becoming the prime object of affection and attachment. These feelings intensify into the Oedipus complex in both sexes, taking on a sexual coloring as the child reaches the phallic stage. The child wishes to possess the mother sexually and is jealous of the father, whom the child views as a rival; a potentially dangerous and destructive situation is usually constructively resolved in the male child by a primary counterforce, castration anxiety.

Castration anxiety is the male child's fear that his father will castrate him if he continues in his decision to possess his mother; when this is reinforced by other losses, the male child is persuaded to give up his "bad" impulses toward his mother. In their place, the boy shifts to an identification with his father, redirecting his sexual intentions to other nonmother feminine objects. During this process of identification, the male introjects his father's value system, forming his own differentiated structure, the superego.

The female child also enters the phallic phase wishing to possess her mother. The child realizes, however, that she has no penis. Feeling betrayed by her sex, she turns to her father whose penis she envies. Initially, she turns toward her father to possess a penis, but as she realizes that this is not possible, she constructs a fantasy world in which she will have her father's child, which she unconsciously equates with the penis.

Beyond this point, the classic psychoanalytic explanation of superego development in the female becomes vague and contradictory. Introjection of the father's values and the formation of the superego through intimidation, general upbringing, and fear of loss of the father's love is the most coherent interpretation. The superego that develops, however, is never as strong as the one developed in the male, leaving the female "showing less sense of justice than men and . . . less ready to submit to the great exigencies of life."[13(p413)]

Neo-Freudian psychoanalytic thought has retained the unitary structure of the superego while reinterpreting the process by which it develops. Klein[18] sees the superego as developing during infancy, with aggression rather than sex being the principle motivation. Most reinterpretations, however, have come from neo-Freudians, who are disturbed at the priority given to biologic rather than societal factors in superego development. Fromm[19] sees the development of the Oedipus complex not as a sexual attraction but rather as a yearning to be free. Horney[20] opposed the theory of penis envy, stating that it was not an envy for a biologic entity but rather for the societal privileges and powers that accompany being male. Miller[21] sees societal influence on superego development resulting in a transformation of the female's drives into the service of others. Finally, Lasch[22] sees society as weakening the structure of the superego so that the aggresive impulses of the id run free.

Cognitive developmental models

For the cognitive developmental models, moral development is the conversion of certain inherent and primitive attitudes and conceptions into a comprehensive set of

For the cognitive developmental models, moral development is the conversion of certain inherent and primitive attitudes and conceptions into a comprehensive set of internal moral standards.

internal moral standards. This conversion process is part of and dependent on the total cognitive growth of individuals as they seek to reorder the social world with which they are continuously interacting.[5] All of the models view this process as a series of stages or patterns of thought that are qualitatively different from each other, constructed through active experience, invariant in order, and the same in sequence for all persons and cultures.

By far the most popular cognitive developmental model has been the one developed by Kohlberg.[23,24] Relying initially on a two-stage model developed by Piaget and on Piaget's view of justice as the core of morality, Kohlberg developed a three-level model of moral development with two stages at each level (see boxed material).

In the testing of Kohlberg's model, one recurring phenomenon was the apparent stage arrest of the overwhelming majority of females at level II, stage 3. For Kohlberg, cognitive development is a process of reordering the social world; its arrest at stage 3 reflects the state of interaction of the female and her social world. The provocation for moving to the next higher stage in the model is the cognitive disequilibrium initiated by the present stage's increasing inability to adequately resolve current moral dilemmas.

As long as females feel that they are adequately resolving their moral dilemmas at the lower stage, Kohlberg felt they

---

Cognitive-Development Model (Kohlberg)

Level I, preconventional morality: Level of morality in which the perspective is egocentric.
   Stage 1, heteronomous morality: Right is might, the reason for doing right is to avoid punishment by those with superior power.
   Stage 2, instrumental morality: Right is following rules when it is to someone's immediate interest; acting to meet one's own interest and needs and letting others do the same. Right is also what is fair, what is an equal exchange, a deal, or an agreement.
Level II, conventional morality: Level of morality in which the perspective is societal.
   Stage 3, mutual morality: Right is living up to what is expected or what people generally expect of people in a certain role. "Being good" is important and means having good motives, showing concern for and about others, and keeping mutual relationships, such as trust, loyalty, respect, and gratitude.
   Stage 4, social system morality: Right is fulfilling the actual duties agreed on. Laws are to be upheld except in extreme cases where they conflict with other fixed social duties. Right is also contributing to society, the group, or the institution.
Level III, postconventional morality: Level of morality in which the perspective is universal.
   Stage 5, social contract morality: Right is being aware that people hold a variety of values and opinions, and that most values and rules are relative to the groups'. These relative rules would usually be upheld, however, in the interest of impartiality and because they are the social contract. Some nonrelative values and rights such as life and liberty, however, must be upheld in any society and regardless of majority opinion.
   Stage 6, universal ethical (principled) morality: Right is following self-chosen ethical principles. Particular laws or social agreements are usually valid because they rest on such principles. When laws violate these principles, one acts in accordance with the principle. Principles are universal principles of justice, the equality of human rights, and respect for the dignity of human beings as individuals.

would never proceed up the model. Kohlberg did think, however, that women's development could proceed beyond this stage when "they are challenged to solve moral problems that require them to see beyond the relationships that in the past have generally bound their moral experience."[25(p323)]

This stage arrest was interpreted differently, however, by Gilligan.[4,26] She argued that instead of being deviant or arrested, feminine moral development was simply, but importantly, different from masculine moral development. She agreed with Kohlberg that both females and males developed their moral judgment in conjunction with their social interaction. However, since the interaction differed between the sexes, the moral stages that resulted were different. Due to their lack of power and the resulting dependence females shared with each other and their children in a male-dominated culture, Gilligan felt that females have had to develop a sense of responsibility based on the universal principle of caring to survive.

Gilligan's resulting model has three levels with two transitional states (see boxed material). As with other cognitive developmental models, the orientation of the individual moves from egocentric to society to universal.

Social learning model

Whereas the cognitive developmental model looks primarily to internal influences for moral development, the social learning model looks to societal influences. Social learning theory views all behavior, including moral behavior, as learned.[27-29]

Moral development is the learning

Cognitive–Developmental Model (Gilligan)

Level I, orientation to individual survival: Morality is sanctions imposed by society. Being moral is surviving by being submissive to authority. The perspective is egocentric.
Transition from selfishness to responsibility. Responsibility for and to others is more important than surviving through submission.
Level II, goodness as self-sacrifice: Goodness is viewed as relying on shared norms or expectations. Being moral is first of all and above all not hurting others, with no thought of the hurt that might be done to self.
Transition from goodness to truth. Responsibility for not hurting others shifts to include not only others, but self.
Level III, morality of nonviolence: The injunction against hurting becomes the moral principle governing all moral judgements. This injunction includes an equality of self and others. Care, instead of individual rights, becomes the universal obligation.

---

process by which specific types of competencies, ie, skills, rules, and cognitive capacities, are acquired for possible use in generating certain types of behavior. Humans, especially children, are constantly observing the behavior that surrounds them. From the social learning perspective, we are all models of behavior for each other. Through the cognitive sensory process, a great deal of information is actively stored away in cognitive constructions, creating large potentials for generating organized behavior.

Whether these potential behaviors are actually performed depends on reinforcement but not just the mere existence of such reinforcement. Additionally, in the moral situation, behavior performance depends first on the person's expectancies or the possibility held by the individual that a particular reinforcement will occur.[30] Second, the occurrence of that reinforcement depends on the individual's subjective values or the degree of a person's preference. And finally, it depends on the individual's inner control, or rather, the contingency rules which guide that individual's behavior in the absence of, and sometimes in spite of, immediate reinforcements.[31]

In the learning process that is moral development, as with others, people, especially parents, vary in what they model and reinforce in children of differing ages. Initially, in the nonverbal child, control is external. Parents provide physical intervention to keep the child from hazardous situations. As the child matures, social sanctions gradually replace the physical ones. As the cognitive structures multiply and mature, there is a gradual substitution of external sanctions and demands for symbolic and internal control. After the moral standards are established by cognition and modeling, self-evaluative consequences serve as deterrents to transgressive acts. As the child grows older and the nature and seriousness of possible transgressions change, parents alter their moral reasoning, moving from individual implications of the acts for the individual child to legalistic, societal arguments.[28]

EVALUATION OF MODELS

Consideration and implementation of any model of moral development by nursing should not occur until an evaluation process with well-delineated criteria has been completed. In the present evaluation, the criteria to be used are empiric relevance, intersubjectivity, and usefulness.

Empiric relevance

Empiric relevance is the process of comparing some aspect of the model with objective empiric research and then determining the congruence between the model's claims and the existing empiric evidence. It is the tightness of this fit that determines the confidence given to any theory or model. And it is often this criterion that determines whether the claim should be considered scientific knowledge.[32]

Psychoanalytic model

Clinical case studies have provided the preponderance of the validation for the psychoanalytic model of superego development.[33,34] Such case studies with their subjective analysis do not, however, constitute empiric testing.[35] The results of objective research have either been questionable or have not supported the model. Katcher,[36] following up on two earlier studies,[37,38] found that half of the children at the Oedipal age are not fully aware of the genital anatomic differences that are supposed to be so traumatic, and therefore, crucial to their superego development.

Freud's conceptualization of the superego as a unified entity has been the basis for the hypothesis that persons of high moral character would display that character in all moral situations. Resulting studies[39,40] have, however, found that there is only a low consistency between the moral behavior of an individual in many different types of moral situations. Supporters of the unitary superego have rebutted these studies with theoretic arguments of ego mediation (explanation of this inconsistent behavior by the mediating effect of the ego on the superego)[41] and with arguments of islands of superego (free-floating islands that at times affect moral behavior and at other times do not).[42] The proponents of these arguments have, however, given no indication how these arguments would be operationalized for an objective empiric research study.

Still other authors have proposed the hypothesis that the stronger a child's fear of the father, the greater the resulting moral standards.[43] Some studies have, however, indicated the opposite:[44-46] that highly nurturing, loving fathers are correlated to sons with high moral standards. In one study, this positive correlation occurred only when the father was the dominant parent.[45] Finally, if the model is valid, a stronger superego could be predicted in males. Hall[47] hypothesized that the weaker superego in females would have more difficulty holding back the aggressive impulses of the id.[47]

Although he affirmed his hypothesis, the results are still questionable, for his method of data analysis was symbolic dream interpretation, and the interpreter was a psychoanalytic therapist who was also a male. The conclusion reached from the available objective research is that the psychoanalytic model has little empiric relevance.

Cognitive–developmental models

Empiric relevance for the cognitive-developmental model of Kohlberg is controvertible. Kohlberg[5] felt that he had validated the invariant order of his stages by retesting his subjects at 3-year intervals. Others testing at 1- to 4-year intervals also

felt they had confirmed this claim.[48,49] The claim has been challenged, however, by researchers who found regression among young adults at the higher stages.[50,51] Kohlberg and his colleagues have had a difficult time explaining a recurrent regression by adolescents from stage 4 to what appear to be stage 2 type moral judgments. They finally developed, but never completely operationalized, a new stage $4\frac{1}{2}$ to account for this phenomenon.[52]

Kohlberg[53] felt that cross-cultural studies validated his assertion that the model is universal to all humans, regardless of culture or religion. He claims that data gathered in Taiwan, Great Britain, Mexico, Turkey, and the United States support this position. Simpson[54] challenges this claim, however, citing vague and unverifiable analogies between Mexicans and American blacks, use of culturally biased data-gathering techniques, and the inability of the research to account for all of the findings. Recent studies have supported Simpson's claim of cultural bias[55] and have indicated that religion may play more of a role in moral judgment than Kohlberg previously recognized.[56]

Another issue of empiric relevance is the test instrument used by Kohlberg to determine the level of moral judgment. Kohlberg has always used a set of hypothetical moral dilemmas followed by open-ended questioning.[5,23,25]

Sensitive to early criticism that the explanations of test procedures were vague and contradictory,[51,54] Kohlberg published his most comprehensive description of the tool and its development. He revealed that three different versions of the tool have been used from the time of the initial study to the present. Agreement among raters, at least in the second version, was 90% in the hands of *thoroughly trained* and *experienced* scorers.[23] Test-retest reliability has not been strong for any of the versions.[57] None of the literature mentions the possibility of action being taken to control for differences in the scoring of any one individual, if different versions of the test were used at different testing sessions.

Another cognitive developmental researcher, Rest, has developed an objective type test for stage identification. Initially, the correlation between Rest's Defining Issues Test (DIT) and Kohlberg's tool (with no identification of which version of Kohlberg's tool was used) was 0.68.[49,57-59] More recent researchers[60,61] have, however, found correlations as low as 0.24 and only as high as 0.41. In addition, both Rest and Kohlberg have indicated that the two tests may be testing different phenomen. Rest considers his test to be more of a recognition exercise, probably resulting in a higher percentage of stage 5 and stage 6 scores.[49,59] Additionally, Kohlberg states explicitly that Rest's DIT is "not useful for testing theoretical propositions from the cognitive developmental theory of moral development."[23(p46)]

Another concern of empiric relevance is Kohlberg's claim that the moral stage is positively correlated with moral behavior.[23] Several nurse researchers who have used Kohlberg's model have made recommendations to nursing eduction, service, and research based on this claim.[8,62-66] A comprehensive review of the studies that attempted to validate this claim yielded only low correlations.[67] There was some variation, however, in the strength of the correlations between levels of moral judgment and moral behavior, depending on the outcome criteria used; ie, there was more support for the claim that individuals with higher moral stage tended to be more honest than for the claim that individuals at higher stages of moral reasoning resist more than others the social pressure to conform in their moral action.

It is apparent that the empiric relevance of Kohlberg's model is still in the process of being tested. Sufficient empiric relevance can be substantiated to give the model potential use for nursing. This model is the only one being implemented by nurse researchers in investigating the moral development and reasoning of both students and practitioners.[8,62-66,68] The concern is not that the model is being implemented but that few of the limitations of the model have been identified by these authors. This is not to indicate that these researchers should destroy their theoretic framework before they begin but rather that the limitations should be discussed so that the consumers of this research are more fully informed.

Social learning model

Empiric relevance of the social learning model as a cohesive whole has not been substantial. The greatest number of research studies have focused on the role of modeling or observations in the learning experience that is moral development. Such studies have demonstrated that the changes in moral behavior initiated by observation of modeling cues are often maintained over time.[69-71] Studies seeking to determine under what conditions modeling is most likely to occur have indicated that what others observe a model doing is more likely to be imitated than are instructions, either written or verbal.[72,73] Finally, the impact of the personal attributes of the model has been examined. Models who are viewed as nurturing or competent and models who are viewed as having higher social status are most likely to be imitated.[74-76] The studies questioning the claim that the stricter the parent, the higher the moral standards of the child were a product of the social learning framework.

Although the studies that have used the social learning framework as their theoretic rationale have been carefully done with attention to methodology, it is less clear how those studies fit back into the model. The findings indicate the likelihood of certain behaviors occurring under highly specific circumstances. The effect of these behaviors on the developing cognitive structure of the individual is less clear. What determines whether these behaviors will develop cognitive structures? How do performances, preferences, or comprehensive deficits affect this cognitive structure? Furthermore, none of the studies have spoken to the effects of multiple divergent modeling cues, by either the same model or differing ones, a situation that is far more common in the social world in which we interact daily.

Intersubjectivity

Intersubjectivity translates as a description in necessary detail, with terms selected so that the audience agrees on their meanings. It includes the use of logical systems that are shared and accepted by relevant scientists.[32]

The psychoanalytic model rates well in intersubjectivity. Terms used to describe the process of superego development are well defined (see boxed material). These terms have become so familiar that they have been incorporated into our daily rhetoric ("Freudian slips"). It is possible to follow the explanation of the process from infancy to Oedipus complex, castration anxiety, identification with the father's values, and differentiation of the superego, at least in males. The logical rigor of the process is, however, problematic for females whose resulting structure is left less well differentiated (see Fig 1).

The cognitive–developmental models

None of the studies have spoken to the effects of multiple divergent modeling cues, by either the same model or differing ones, a situation that is far more common in the social world in which we interact daily.

Psychoanalytic Concepts

Castration anxiety: Fear of castration, which induces a repression of sexual desire for the mother and hostility toward the father.

Identification: Method by which a person takes over the features of another person and makes them a corporate part of his or her own personality.

Introjection: Mechanism by which the superego is incorporated into the personality; to take in.

Oedipus complex: Sexual attraction for the parent of the opposite sex and hostility toward the parent of the same sex.

Penis envy: Discovery by the female of the absence of the penis and the subsequent desire to possess the penis she lacks.

Phallic stage: 3rd stage of personality development during which the sexual and aggressive feelings associated with the function of the genitals comes into focus.

Superego: Part of the personality that represents the moral standards of society as conveyed to a person by his or her parents.

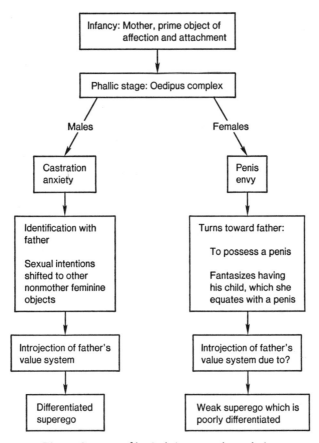

Fig 1. Systems of logical rigor: psychoanalytic.

also rate well in intersubjectivity. In both Kohlberg's and Gilligan's models, terms are well defined and used uniformly in all of the literature. Furthermore, the logical systems of both models are comprehended readily without undue strife. The progress from egocentric to societal to universal is explained in detail in both models (see Figs 2 and 3).

The social learning model rates well in the description of terms but less favorably in the use of a logical system. (See boxed material.) Although terms are well defined in individual studies, how these terms and the behaviors they represent fit back into

the model is frequently in question. Does the learning that occurs from modeling become cognitions, which are potential behaviors, or reinforcers? Does learning strengthen expectancies, subjective values, or both? These are just a few of the questions that the model raises but does not clarify (see Fig 4).

Usefulness

Usefulness, the utility of the model in explaining or controlling the phenomena of interest, is considered by some to be the ultimate test for significance.[77] Whether a model is useful for nurses who wish to

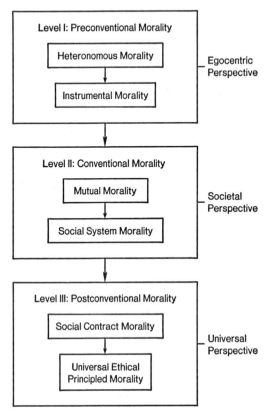

Fig 2. Systems of logical rigor: cognitive-developmental, Kohlberg.

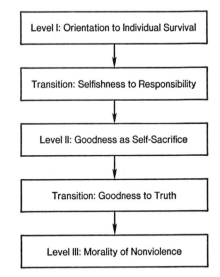

Fig 3. Systems of logical rigor: cognitive-developmental, Gilligan.

implement a model of moral development in education, practice, or research is contingent on the confidence they have in the model. This confidence is ultimately a reflection of how well the model has fared in its empiric relevance and intersubjectivity. Table 1 shows the comparative usefulness of the models.

FURTHER CONSIDERATIONS

Most professions have recognized that their responsibility in preparing and assisting morally competent practitioners is not finished with the publication of codes of

---

Social Learning Concepts

Behavior: Performance

Cognitive construction (competencies): Behavioral repertoire and skills in processing information developed through observational learning and direct experience.

Contingency rules: Guide behavior in absence of and sometimes in spite of immediate situational pressures.

Expectancies: Possibility held by individual that a particular reinforcement will occur.

Imitation: Response mimicry of observed behavior.

Modeling: Observation of an unusual set of responses performed by another individual.

Potential behaviors: Reception, organization, and storing of information that is available for performance.

Reinforcements: Consequence that produces a decrease or increase in repetition of a behavior.

Subjective values: Degree of a person's preference for that reinforcement.

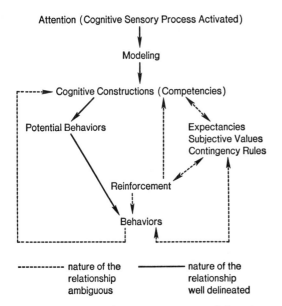

Attention (Cognitive Sensory Process Activated)

Modeling

Cognitive Constructions (Competencies)

Potential Behaviors

Expectancies
Subjective Values
Contingency Rules

Reinforcement

Behaviors

---------- nature of the
relationship
ambiguous

———— nature of the
relationship
well delineated

Fig 4. Systems of logical rigor: social learning theory.

conduct. Although such codes are undeniably beneficial, they are not sufficient for generating morally responsible professionals. To be propitious, these codes must be implemented both intentionally and appropriately by the individual health care pro-

fessional. The process that any profession, including nursing, implements to actualize such professional practitioners should not depend on speculation and chance. Rather, the process of producing such morally competent health care professionals should be intentional, grounded on an identified model of moral development. It should not be decided haphazardly which model or combination of models that nursing implements; this should be decided deliberately following due consideration.

The primary consideration should be, of course, the robustness of the model as evaluated by delineated criteria. This evaluation should not be, however, the only consideration. Other concerns, usually arising from the primary one, need to be recognized and evaluated.

One such consideration for nursing is the congruency of the chosen model of moral development with other theoretic frameworks being used by the setting. Each of the moral development models is based on certain assumptions about the

Table 1. Usefulness of models

| Model | Empiric relevance | Intersubjectivity | |
		Description of terms	System of logical rigor
Psychoanalytic	Little empiric support	Terms well delineated	Adequate for males Ambiguous for females
Cognitive-developmental	Studies have both confirmed and disavowed Kohlberg's models	Terms well delineated	Logical system well delineated
Social learning	Studies are well done, although the nature of their relationship to the model is often ambiguous	Terms well delineated	Nature of relationships ambiguous

nature of humans. Nursing's theoretic frameworks are also based on such assumptions. Choice of a model of moral development should not occur until the assumptions underlying both the moral model and the nursing framework have been identified and compared. If the profession is serious regarding its efforts to develop or support a morally competent professional, it seems detrimental to implement a model of moral development that views the human as an organism that is seeking equilibrium with an environment separate from the self,[78] whereas the model of nursing practice being implemented views humans as coextensive with the universe.[79]

When a moral development mode is chosen for implementation another exigent consideration for nursing is that the great majority of the members of the profession are females. All of the models recognize that moral development is different in males and females. This difference is complicated in several of the models, however, by the preferential perspective given by males to the masculine dimensions inherent in the models. The classic psychoanalytic model saw feminine moral development and the end product or superego as ambiguous. Although the superego could be strengthened through the transference that occurred during psychoanalytic therapy, ultimately, by virtue of her anatomy, the female was limited in the process she could perform in differentiating her superego.

Kohlberg, who is a male, developed his model using only male subjects. When females were consistently at one level, he demanded that they modify themselves to fit the masculine standard, which he viewed as superior. The alternative option that the model might need to be modified or expanded has never been a serious consideration for Kohlberg. Finally, the social learning model sees the differences as resulting from the different learning experiences of males and females. For this model, the differences result from the socialization process and have less of a value dimension than do the differences in the preceding models.

USE OF MORAL DEVELOPMENT MODELS BY NURSING

Kohlberg's cognitive developmental model of moral development is by far the most popular model in nursing currently. The only published nursing research studies in moral development have been based on Kohlberg's model.[8,62-66,68] In addition, at least one curriculum in nursing is using the model.[80] Its popularity and subsequent use probably has several causes. The model is easily operationalized by nursing for nursing research. And it is an optimistic one, promising moral development as an inevitable process, if the health care professional is exposed to appropriate role models when faced with cognitive disequilibrium.

Influence of the other models has been less direct. Many discussions of ethical decision making in the nursing literature speak of reinforcers or of the positive or negative consequences of a set of behaviors,[81-84] using the terminology of social learning theory. The authors do not, however, explicitly acknowledge that these models are based in the social learning framework. The influence of the psychoanalytic model is even less readily apparent. Each time, however, a nurse counsels either a fellow professional or a client, with her goal being the identification of unconscious motivators to moral behavior, she is basing her intervention on the psychoanalytic model.

Nursing is just beginning to explore the variables that interact to account for moral thinking and behavior. The profession has only just begun to explore the process by which we can expedite more principled thinking in ourselves and in the client. This exploration must continue if we are to facilitate the professional nurse who is increasingly faced with health care situations that call for moral judgments.

REFERENCES

1. Plato: Meno, in Rouse WHD (translator): *Great Dialogues of Plato*. New York, New American Library, 1956, pp. 28-68.
2. Dock S: The relationship of the nurse to the doctor and the doctor to the nurse. *Am J Nurs* 1917;17:394.
3. Murphy CP: The moral situation in nursing, in Bandman EL, Bandman B (eds): *Bioethics and Human Rights*. Boston, Little Brown & Co, 1978, pp 313-320.
4. Gilligan C: In a different voice: Women's conception of self and morality. *Harvard Educ Rev* 1977;17:482-517.
5. Kohlberg L: The development of children's orientation toward a moral order: I. Sequence in the development of moral thought. *Vita Humana* 1963;6:11-33.
6. Shiveder RA, Turiel E, Much NC: The moral institutions of the child, in Flavell J, Ross L (eds): *Social Cognitive Development*. Cambridge, England, Cambridge University Press, 1981, pp 288-305.
7. Thiroux JP: *Ethics*. Beverly Hills, Calif, Glencoe Press, 1977.
8. Kudzma EA: *Moral Reasoning of Nurses in the Work Setting*, doctoral dissertation. Boston University School of Nursing, May 1980.
9. Thompson JB, Thompson HD: *Ethics in Nusing*. New York, Macmillan Publishing Co Inc, 1981.
10. Beauchamp TL, Childress JF: *Principles of Bioethics*. New York, Oxford University Press, 1979.
11. Chazan BI: The moral situation, in Soltis JF, Chazan BI (eds): *Moral Education*. New York, Teacher's College Press, 1973, pp 39-49.
12. Freud S: *The Ego and the Id*. New York, WW Norton & Co Inc, 1960.
13. Freud S: Some physical consequences of the anatomical distinction between the sexes, in *The Standard Edition of the Works of Sigmund Freud*. London, Hogarth Press, 1961, vol 19, pp 413-425.
14. Freud S: *New Introductory Lectures on Psychoanalysis*. New York, WW Norton & Co Inc, 1965.
15. Freud S: *Outline of Psychoanalysis*. New York, WW Norton & Co Inc, 1960.
16. Freud S: The dissolution of the Oedipus complex, in Mischel HN, Mischel W (eds): *Readings in Personality*. New York, Holt Rinehart & Winston Inc, 1973, pp 90-95.
17. Hall CS: *A Primer of Freudian Psychology*. New York, The New American Library Inc, 1979.
18. Klein M: *The Psychoanalysis in Children*. New York, Delta Books, 1975.
19. Fromm E: *Man for Himself: An Inquiry into the Psychology of Ethics*. Greenwich, Conn, Fawcett Publications Inc, 1947.
20. Horney K: *Feminine Psychology*. New York, WW Norton & Co Inc, 1967.
21. Miller JB: *Toward a New Psychology for Women*. Boston, Beacon Press, 1976.
22. Lasch C: *The Culture of Narcissism*. New York, WW Norton & Co Inc, 1979.
23. Kohlberg L: Moral stages and moralization: The cognitive-development approach, in Lilkona T (ed): *Moral Development: Theory, Research, and Social Issues*. New York, Holt Rinehart & Winston Inc, 1976, pp 31-53.
24. Kohlberg L: *Essays on Moral Development: The Philosophy of Moral Development*. Cambridge, Mass, Harper & Row Publishers, Inc, 1981.
25. Kohlberg L: From is to ought: How to commit the naturalistic fallacy and get away with it in the study of moral development, in Mischel T (ed): *Cognitive Development and Epistemology*. New York, Academic Press, 1971, pp 151-235.
26. Gilligan C: Women's place in a man's life cycle. *Harvard Educ Rev* 1979;19:432-446.
27. Bandura A, Walters RH: *Social Learning and Person-*

ality Development. New York, Holt Rinehart and Winston Inc, 1963.

28. Bandura A: *Social Learning Theory*. Englewood Cliffs, NJ, Prentice-Hall Inc, 1977.

29. Rohrbaugh JB: *Women: Psychology's Puzzle*. New York, Basic Books Inc, 1979.

30. Rotter JB, Chance J, Phares EJ: An introduction to social learning theory, in Mischel HN, Mischel W (eds): *Readings in Personality*. New York, Holt Rinehart and Winston Inc, 1973, pp 148-151.

31. Mischel W, Mischel HN: A cognitive social learning appproach to morality and self-regulation, in Lilkona T (ed): *Moral Development and Behavior: Theory, Research, and Social Issues*. New York, Holt Rinehart & Winston Inc, 1976, pp 84-107.

32. Reynolds PD: *A Primer in Theory Construction*. Indianapolis, Bobbs-Merrill Co Inc, 1971.

33. Furer M: The history of the superego concept psychoanalysis: A review of the literature, in Post S (ed): *Moral Value and the Superego Concept in Psychoanalysis*. New York, International Universities Press, 1972, pp 11-62.

34. Carrington P, Harmon SE: Moral consideration in the psychotherapy of an adolescent who attempted murder, in Seymour P (ed): *Moral Values and the Superego Concept in Psychoanalysis*. New York, International Universities Press, 1972, pp 156-167.

35. Hardy ME: Perspectives on nursing theory. *Adv Nurs Sci* 1978;1(1):37-48.

36. Katcher A: The discrimination of sex differences by young children. *J Genet Psychol* 1955;87:131-143.

37. Conn JH: Children's reactions to the discovery of genital differences. *Am J Orthopsychiatry* 1940;10:747-754.

38. Conn JH, Kramer L: Children's awareness of sex differences. *J Child Psychiatry* 1947;1:3-57.

39. Hartshorne H, May MA: *Studies in the Nature of Character*. New York, Macmillan, 1930.

40. Fischer S, Greenberg RP: *The Scientific Credibility of Freud's Theories and Therapy*. New York, Basic Books, 1977.

41. Kline P: *Fact and Fantasy in Freudian Theory*. London, Methuen & Co Ltd, 1972.

42. Redl F, Wineman D: *The Aggressive Child*. New York, Free Press, 1955.

43. Bettleheim B: Moral education, in Sizer T (ed): *Moral Education: Five Lectures*. Cambridge, Mass, Harvard University Press, 1970, pp 85-107.

44. Hoffman M: Child-rearing practices and moral development: Generalizations from empirical research. *Child Dev* 1963;34:295-318.

45. Moulton RW, Liberty PG, Burnstein E, Altucher N: Patterning of parental affection and discipline as a determinant of guilt and sex typing. *J Pers Soc Psychol* 1966;4:356-363.

46. Unger SM: Antecedents of personality difference sin guilt responsitivity. *Psychol Rep* 1962;10:357, 358.

47. Hall CS: A modest confirmation of Freud's theory of a distinction between the superego of men and women. *J Psychol* 1964;69:440-442.

48. Kuhn D: Short term longitudinal evidence for the sequence of Kohlberg's stages of moral development. *Dev Psychol* 1976;12:162-166.

49. Rest JR, Davidson ML, Robbin S: Age trends in judging moral issues: A review of cross-sectional, longitudinal, and sequential studies of the defining issues test. *Child Dev* 1978;49:263-279.

50. Holstein CB: Irreversible, stepwise sequence in the development of moral judgement: A longitudinal study of males and females. *Child Dev* 1976;47:51-61.

51. Kurtines W, Grief EB: The development of moral thought: Review and explanation of Kohlberg's approach. *Psychol Bull* 1974;81:453-470.

52. Gilligan C, Kohlberg L: From adolescence to adulthood: The discovery of reality in a post-conventional world, in Presseisen B, Goldman D, Appel MH (eds): *Topics in Cognitive Development*. New York, Plenum Press, 1978, pp 125-136.

53. Kohlberg L: Education for justice: A modern statement of the platonic view, in Sizer T (ed): *Moral Education: Five Lectures*. Cambridge, Mass, Harvard University Press, 1970, pp 57-83.

54. Simpson EL: Moral development research: A case study of cultural bias. *Hum Dev* 1974;17:81-106.

55. Harkeess S, Edwards CP. Super CM: Social roles and moral reasoning: A study in a rural African community. *Dev Psychol* 1981;17:595-601.

56. Erndierger DJ, Manaster GJ: Moral development, intrinsic/extrinsic religious orientation and denominational teachings. *Genet Psychol Monogr* 1981;104:23-41.

57. Rest JR: Recent research in an objective test of moral judgement: How the important issues of a moral dilema are defined, in DePalma DJ, Foley JM (eds): *Moral Development: Current Theory and Research*. New York, John Wiley & Sons, 1975, pp 75-93.

58. Rest JR: New approaches in the assessment of moral judgement, in Lilkona T (ed): *Moral Development and Behavior: Theory, Research, and Social Issues*. New York, Holt Rinehart & Winston, 1976, pp 198-218.

59. Rest JR: Longitudinal study of the Defining Issues Test. *Dev Psychol* 1975;11:738-749.

60. Bode J, Page R: Comparisons of measures of moral development. *Psychol Rep* 1978;43:307-312.

61. Davidson D, Robbins S: The reliability and validity

of objective indices of moral development. *App Psychol Measurement* 1978;2:389-401.

62. Ketefian S: Critical thinking. Educational program and development of moral judgement among selected groups of practicing nurses. *Nurs Res* 1981;30:98-103.

63. Ketefian S: Moral reasoning and moral behavior among selected groups of practicing nurses: Part II. *Nurs Res* 1981;30:171-176.

64. Mahon K, Fowler MO: Moral development and clinical decision making. *Nurs Clin North Am* 1978;14:3-12.

65; Munhall P: Moral reasoning levels of nursing students and faculty in a baccalaureate nursing program. *Image* 1980;12:57-61.

66. Murphy C: Moral reasoning in a select group of nursing practitioners, in Ketefian S (ed): *Perspectives on Nursing Leadership*. New York, Teacher's College Press, 1981, pp 45-76.

67. Blasi A: Bridging moral cognition and moral action: A critical review of the literature. *Psychol Bull* 1980;88:1-45.

68. Crisham P: Measuring moral judgement in moral dilemmas. *Nurs Res* 1980;30:104-110.

69. Bandura A: Influence of model's reinforcement contingencies on the acquisition of imitative behaviors. *J Pers Soc Psychol* 1965;1:589-595.

70. Bandura A; Ross D, Ross SA: Vicarious reinforcement and imitative learning. *Journal Abnorm Soc Psychol* 1963;67:601-607.

71. Bandura A, McDonald FJ: Influence of social reinforcement and the behavior of models in shaping children's moral judgements. *J Abnorm Soc Psychol* 1963;67:274-281.

72. Mischel W, Tiebert RM: Effects of discrepancies between observed and imposed reward criteria on the acquisition and transmission of behavior. *J Pers Soc Psychol* 1966;3:45-53.

73. Bryan JH: You will be advised to watch what we do instead of what we say, in DePalma J, Foley JM (eds): *Moral Dev: Curr Theory Res.* John Wiley & Sons, 1975, pp 95-112.

74. Lefkowitz M, Blake RR, Moulton JS: Status factors in pedestrian violations of traffic signals. *J Abnorm Soc Psychol* 1955;51;704-705.

75. Grusec J, Mischel W: Model's characteristics and determinants of social learning. *J Pers Soc Psychol* 1966;4;211-215.

76. Baron RA: Attraction toward the model and model's competence as determinants of adult imitative behaviors. *J Pers Soc Psychol* 1970;14:345-351.

77. Ellis R: Characteristics of significant theories. *Nurs Res* 1968;17:268-274.

78. Kohlberg L: Stage and sequence: The cognitive developmental approach to socialization, in Goslin D (ed): *Handbook of Socialization Theory and Research.* Chicago, Rand McNally, 1969, pp 329-395.

79. Rogers M: *An Introduction to the Theoretical Basis of Nursing.* Philadelphia, FA Davis Co, 1970.

80. Johnston T: Moral education for nursing. *Nurs Forum* 1980;14:284-299.

81. Andrews S, Hutchinson SA: Teaching nursing ethics: A practical approach. *J Nurs Educ* 1981;20:6-16.

82. Curtin L: A proposed model for critical ethical analysis. *Nurs Forum* 1978;17:4-11.

83. Heynes KM: An ethical decision system, in Davis AJ, Kreuger J (eds): *Patients, Nurses, Ethics.* New York, American Journal of Nursing Co, 1980, pp 9-21.

84. Ryden M: An approach to ethical decision making. *Nurs Outlook* 1978;26:705-706.

The Politics of Medical Deception: Challenging the Trajectory of History

Mariann C. Lovell, R.N.
Master's Candidate
Wright State University
Dayton, Ohio

THE RELATIONSHIPS between medicine and nursing and between nurses, patients and physicians have historically been symbiotic. Medicine has carefully nurtured this symbiosis with calculated deception, paternalistic hostility and blatant sexism. The economic, political and social forces inherent in these practices have been systematically manipulated by the medical profession throughout the past century. As the United States embarks on the 1980s, these abuses continue to enhance medicine's power and control over people's minds and bodies. Although it may be painful for nurses to acknowledge that their personal and professional identities have been dictated and diminished by others, such an acknowledgment must be made if nurses are to stop these

This article is based on research completed for "An Historical Study of the Development of the Medical Profession as a Business: Impact on Nursing and Society, 1896-1979," master's thesis, Wright State University, Dayton, Ohio, 1980.

abuses and enter into a politics of care that is not encumbered by deception.

THE OPPRESSIVE POLITICS OF MEDICINE

Many writers claim that the health care system is intimately associated with politics,[1,2] but few are willing to admit that politics is also an integral part of interactions with physicians, whether client-physician interactions or nurse-physician interactions. Power is presently being used by the medical profession against the interests of nursing and society, yet most people are only dimly aware of what is going on. This lack of awareness, combined with a reluctance to question what is not understood, renders nursing and society powerless.

Political thinking among physicians in the United States can be traced to the origins of the American medical profession itself. As early as the 1830s, medicine endeavored to enhance their economic rewards. At that time the "regular doctors"—the professional ancestors of today's physicians—were outnumbered by the "irregulars" who emphasized preventive care and health education of the public. Because of the preventive nature of irregular practice, as opposed to the "murderous cures" and "radical elitism" espoused by the regular doctors, popular support remained with the former.[3,4] Women and members of the working class were especially vocal in their support of the irregulars. To circumvent future competition by irregulars, medicine (the regulars) attempted to set themselves up as the undisputed "real doctors."[5]

This attempt to become the only recognized doctors propelled the onslaught of political maneuvering among physicians. The initial failure to establish a medical monopoly via mandatory medical licensure during the early 1840s merely intensified physicians' political orientation.[6] This early failure to achieve control made it clear that although a great deal of money could be made in medicine, more attention must be paid to the economic concepts of supply, demand and competition. It was recognized that to accomplish this economic goal, social and political forces must be carefully controlled. Medical efforts in this direction commenced in 1847 when the regular doctors pulled together their first national organization, the American Medical Association (AMA).[7]

One of the politician's first principles is to avoid taking on any more organized opposition than is necessary. The first principle for those who want to influence politicians is to organize. With this elementary rule in mind, millions of people have banded together in some 2,000 organizations and sent their men to Washington to lobby for their special interest groups. By far the most powerful and resolute legislative lobby in Washington is the AMA.[8(p322), 9(p1)] Indeed one of the historic purposes of organizing medicine in 1847 was to influence governmental decisions.[8(p321)] The AMA did not acquire internal unity until the late 1800s and did not attain real strength until direct hierarchical authority (from local through county and state to the national level) was established in 1902. Until then the association had no real power on a national scale.[6]

The medical offensive thrust to capture a legal monopoly over the practice of medicine was fortified with Flexner's report on medical education reform.[4,6] As a direct result of the methodical medical maneuverings that culminated in the Flexner report, most states ruled that practicing medicine without a license was a crime punishable by prison confinement. A legal monopoly was thus established, and the AMA heralded its intent to maintain power and control.[6]

Having achieved control over entry into the profession via licensure, artificially high standards and certification rules, the AMA devoted more of its energies and considerable resources to persuading any-

---

Prior to World War I the AMA became an effective, organized political action group working primarily for physicians' economic interests.

---

one who would listen, particularly lawmakers, that the only way to bring about the betterment of public health was to keep it in private hands. The organized medical profession won its first major political battle against national health insurance in this pre-World War I era. In doing so the AMA became an effective, organized political action group working primarily for physicians' economic interests.[7,8] Harris aptly illustrates the power and control wielded by organized medicine during its 45-year, multimillion-dollar fight against public health legislation. This blatant commercial pursuit, characteristic of medical practice since its formal incep-

tion in this country,[9] has led the AMA to oppose even the mildest and most constructive official and semiofficial intrusions against medicine including:

compulsory inoculation against diphtheria and compulsory vaccination against smallpox, the mandatory reporting of tuberculosis cases to public-health agencies, the establishment of public venereal-disease clinics and of Red Cross blood banks, federal grants for medical school construction and medical-student loans, Blue Cross and other private health-insurance programs, government subsidies to reduce maternal and infant death, and free centers for cancer diagnosis. The AMA's arguments against these proposals have ranged from charges that they constituted "bureaucratic interference with the sacred right of the American home" to condemnation of them as "tending to promote Communism.[8(p2)]

Olson analyzes why political pressure groups, such as the AMA, command such far-reaching power and control. He theorizes that the lobbies of the large economic groups are the byproducts of organizations that have the capacity to "mobilize" a latent group with "selective incentives." The only organizations that have the selective incentives available are those that have (1) the authority and capacity to be coercive, or (2) a source of positive inducements they can offer the individuals in a latent group.[10(p133)]

This byproduct theory of large pressure groups can be applied at all hierarchical levels of medicine. It is specifically applicable at the level of individual medical practitioners. Physicians, without the power of the AMA, have little incentive to sacrifice their time or money to help an organization obtain a collective good; they alone can rarely be decisive in determining whether or not this collective good will be obtained. But if it is obtained because of the efforts of others the physicians will inevitably be able to enjoy the benefits. Thus they would support the organization with a lobby working for collective goods only if (1) they are coerced into paying dues to the lobbying organization, or (2) they have to support this group in order to obtain some other noncollective benefit. Organized medicine provides both the coercion and the noncollective benefits.

Coercion

Organized medicine has reached for the forbidden fruit of compulsory membership. For a period of time prior to World War II, AMA membership was required to obtain and maintain specialty board certification. Dismissal from the AMA, exclusion for whatever reason (such as lack of social attributes, race, etc.) or unwillingness to join because of conflicting views on the practice of medicine or on attitudes toward compulsory health insurance had a direct bearing on the definition of specialist "merit."[6(p248)] Eventually AMA membership was dropped as a requirement for board certification; membership, however, was strongly "recommended."

V. O. Key argues that the tendency to seek the reality, if not invariably the form, of a guild system is characteristic of the politics of professional associations in general.[10(p137)] The adoption of the guild form of organization supports the byproduct theory of large pressure groups, for a strong leaning toward compulsory membership has always been basic to the guild system. Garceau speaks of the advantages

of maintaining membership and good relationships with a professional association because the recalcitrant physician in trouble with organized medicine may face a genuine economic threat.[11(pp95, 103)]

Noncollective Benefits

The role of coercion, even in its subtler forms in the AMA, is probably less important as a source of membership than the noncollective benefits the organization provides its members. According to Garceau, there is "one formal service of the society with which the doctor can scarcely dispense. Malpractice defense has become a prime requisite to private practice."[11(p103)] Not only is malpractice insurance more expensive for a non-AMA member, but access to other physicians to testify in the physician's behalf during malpractice litigation is severed. Expert witnesses from the ranks of organized medicine are abundantly available for plaintiffs but not for defendants. Therefore the position of the plaintiff in a suit against a nonsociety member is considerably stronger than it is for a suit against a society member.

Other noncollective benefits of AMA membership are the many technical publications of the association and of the state and local medical societies. These offer considerable incentive to affiliate with organized medicine. Since the 19th century *JAMA* has provided "tangible attraction for doctors."[11(p15)] Aside from being the prime money maker of the AMA, gleaning most of its revenue from drug company advertising, *JAMA* serves as the organ through which political information is disseminated. The controlling elements of the AMA are evident in the policy to keep divergent viewpoints on political and economic matters out of the pages of the journal.[12(p171)] *JAMA* has become such a powerful political voice in organized medicine that Morris Fishbein, editor of the publication for nearly 30 years, has been recognized by the public as sole spokesman for American medicine.[12(p175)] As a result, the AMA has been referred to as the American Fishbein Association.[8]

The AMA serves physicians in the capacity of a craft union. It protects and advances the economic interests of its members. The association would have neither the coercive power to exercise nor the noncollective benefits to sell if physicians' economic situations were not so entangled with the politics of control.

Control

Implicit in the definition of coercion is control, domination, intimidation and nullification of individual will.[13(p439)] The coercion the AMA uses on its members is available for members to use to control their patients. Freire explains this phenomenon in terms of oppression theory. The oppressed, having internalized the image of the oppressors and adopted their guidelines, follow prescribed behavior patterns. This prescribed behavior represents the imposition of the oppressors' choice upon the oppressed.[14(pp30,31)] In the situation of medicine, the AMA coerces physicians to conform; physicians in turn coerce their patients, thus modeling themselves after the AMA.

Dehumanization

Another characteristic of oppression attempts to explain the economic basis of medicine's struggle for power and control.

The oppressor consciousness tends to transform everything surrounding it into objects of domination. Everything, including human life, is reduced to the status of objects. Freire describes this unrestrained eagerness to possess:

> ...the oppressors develop the conviction that it is possible for them to transform everything into objects of their purchasing power; hence their strictly materialistic concept of existence. Money is the measure of all things, and profit the primary goal. For the oppressors, what is worthwhile is to have more—always more—even at the cost of the oppressed having less or having nothing. For them, to be is to have and to be the class of the "haves."[14(p44)]

Organized medicine has played an important, even essential, role in profit abuse. Medicine's abuses of profit are not new.[15(p95, 103)] Current concerns about the abuse of women have been poignantly documented by Daly,[3] Rich,[4] and Ehrenreich and English,[16] among others. The theory of innate female sickness, in which medicine "discovered" that female functions were inherently pathological, was skewed so as to account for class differences in ability to pay for medical care. This theory meshed conveniently with the physician's commercial self-interest. Medicine maintained that it was affluent women who were most delicate and most in need of medical attention. Lower class women who were less able to pay for medical care were seen as "blessed" with immunity from uterine disease.[4, 11(p15)] Gilman illuminates the physician's role in this abuse during the late 19th century as she describes S. Weir Mitchell's famous rest cure for affluent women. Women taking this cure had to lie supine in a darkened room for six weeks. They were not permitted to read, write or see anyone except the physician. This cure allegedly allowed the brain to rest so that women could be more feminine.[17] Millett and Chesler report that women continue to be pawns in the business of maximizing profits from illness.[18,19]

The dehumanizing (objectification) element that is the core of oppression theory encompasses violence. Violence is deliberate assault, physical or otherwise, by those who fail to recognize others as fully human. Once an oppressive relationship is established, violence has already begun. Even when the relationship is sweetened by false generosity it remains oppressive because it does not allow for humanness. People become commodities to be used, abused and manipulated at the whim of the oppressor.[14]

POSSESSION, CONTROL AND DECEPTION

Oppressors view themselves as privy to this "thing" called humanity. They possess it as an exclusive right, as inherited property. Constant control of the oppressed becomes necessary to prevent subversion. This phenomenon then becomes cyclical: the more the oppressors control the oppressed, the more the oppressed are changed into inanimate things which in turn require greater control.

Bok adds dimension to the concepts of control and dehumanization. She explores how deception is intricately interwoven with coercion, violence, power and paternalism.[20] Each of these factors can justify the use of deception to control those who have first been objectified. Both deceit

Both deceit and violence can coerce people into acting against their will. But deceit controls more subtly, for it employs belief as well as action.

and violence can coerce people into acting against their will. But deceit controls more subtly, for it employs belief as well as action. When deception is used to coerce it gives power to the deceiver. The power relationship that results, whether it is between physician-patient, physician-nurse, father-child, husband-wife or any two groups or individuals along the medical hierarchy, constitutes oppressive violence because it objectifies and therefore dehumanizes.

Bok defines deception as the intentional communication of messages meant to mislead others. It means making others believe what the deceiver does not believe. Deception can be accomplished through gesture, through disguise, by means of action or inaction, even through silence.[20(p14)] Lying, then, comprises only one small portion of deception: an intentionally deceptive message that is stated (orally or written).

The Silence of History

Rich explores how the silences of history and literature beget powerlessness.[16] The trajectory of history cannot be challenged if the deceptive practices, the secrets, the veiled symbolisms and unasked questions that have served to exploit women, nurses and society remain concealed. The history of nursing and medicine is replete with evidence of medicine's deception and exploitation, of its abuse of women and tacit promotion of disease.[21] A historical analysis of how organized medicine has labored to deceive the public will reveal why nursing and society have allowed this situation to flourish. An understanding of the characteristics basic to deception will provide insight to examine medicine's deceptive practices.

Daly reflects that deception is so totally pervasive in patriarchal society that it is not even named in the traditional listing of the Seven Deadly Sins.[3(p30)] The deception engendered by patriarchy sedates women until their minds and bodies can be controlled and manipulated. Paternalistic lying promotes this female mind sedation by discouraging females from asking questions. So long as questions are unasked, such as when power is thought divinely granted or ordained by nature, the right to coerce and manipulate is taken for granted. When this right is questioned, the answer given by paternalism is that authority is at the very least justified when it is exercised over persons for their own good.[20(p215)]

This type of deception is frequently used for persons of limited understanding such as children, mental incompetents and the uneducated. Individuals bend the truth to convey the "right picture." They believe this will compensate for the inexperience or fears of the listener, just as raising one's voice helps the hard of hearing to understand the message.

Lies can ultimately suffocate and exploit those whom they were ostensibly meant to protect. Bok describes an example:

Throughout history, men, women, and children have been compelled to accept degrading work, alien religious practices, institutionalization, and even wars alleged to "free" them all in the name of what someone has declared to be in their own best interest. And deception may well have outranked force as a means of subjection: duping people to conform . . . [20(p216)]

Political Lies

Political lies differ from other forms of deception in the benefits they may confer and the long-range harm they may avoid. These lies may be broadly paternalistic. The altruistic purposes justifying such lies are mingled with error and self-deception.[20(pp175, 176)] Much deceit for private gain masquerades as being in the public interest. Deception, even for the most unselfish motive, corrupts and spreads.[20] Daly, in her discussion of deception, incorporates the role that myth plays: "Patriarchy perpetuates its deception through myth."[3(p44)] She adds that patriarchal myths contain stolen mythic power because they are phallic distortions of ancient gynocentric civilizations.[3(pp47, 48)]

In American paternalistic society deception is rarely absent from human practices.[20] There are great differences, however, among the professions in this society in the types of deceit that exist and the extent to which deception is practiced. Historical data indicate that organized medicine has carefully cultivated deception throughout its American history. Bok indicates that honesty and truthfulness have been left out altogether from medical oaths and codes of ethics are often ignored in the teaching of medicine.[20(pxvi)] She neglects to mention that the codes of ethics provide fertile ground for a rich harvest of deception.

Code of Ethics

One of the first official acts of the AMA was to adopt a code of ethics at their convention in Philadelphia in May 1847. This document set the tone of commercial pursuit via oppression and deceit that has characterized medical practice since its formal inception in this country. The code of ethics specifically lists the obligations of patients to their physicians: (1) never volunteer information to the physician, just answer the physician's questions; (2) avoid all physicians except your one family physician—do not allow even a friendly visit or pass the time of day with other physicians; and (3) never do anything about your own health care without consulting your physician. The duties of physicians to one another include: (1) do not advertise; and (2) do not offer free advice—not even to the poor. The code of ethics also specified public obligations to physicians: (1) physicians are justly entitled to the utmost consideration and respect, and no amount of money can cancel this "debt"; and (2) physicians are entitled to certain immunity from the law.[22]

Evident in this code of ethics are the rudimentary medical economic policies upon which medical enterprises have been based since the code was established: (1) "ownership" of the patient by the physician; (2) unquestioning patient devotion to one physician; (3) dependence on the physician with resulting loss of confidence in oneself; (4) physician control of information; (5) discouragement of competi-

tion; (6) cultivation of paying clients only; (7) paternalism; and (8) patient belief in the physician's "magic" cures and medicines. Each of these themes contributes to medicine's deceptive exploitation of nursing and society for the purpose of maximizing profits.[9]

The Use of Myth

Medicine's use of myth to promote deception is quite effective. Physicians know only too well how uncertain a diagnosis or prognosis can be. Recovery from illness is as unpredictable as the incidence of the illness. This uncertainty, coupled with the sacred quality that is carefully cultivated in the physician-patient relationship (that is, the patient regards the physician as a god), casts an aura of myth around the selling of medical services. Malinowski explains how myths are related to uncertainty: "Magical beliefs and practices tend to cluster about situations where there is an important uncertainty factor and where there are strong emotional interests in the success of action."[8(p14)]

Aside from religious practices, probably no human situation fits this description better than that of a person purchasing medical services. Parsons expands this concept: "The basic function of magic is to bolster the self-confidence of actors in situations where energy and skill do make a difference but where, because of uncertainty factors, outcomes cannot be guaranteed."[8(p14)] The magical beliefs that arise from the medical situation are projected onto the physician. Bressler believes that physicians unconsciously regard themselves as magicians and come to partially accept the public view of their infallibility.[23(pp26, 27)]

The image of physicians as infallible gods and magicians did not evolve unassisted. The current symbol for the medical profession, the caduceus, was officially chosen in the 16th century. It shows the wand of Mercury, messenger of the gods and himself the god of dreams, magic and trade.[24] Medicine has carefully cultivated and capitalized on this image. Physicians are priests/gods and as such are entitled to reverence, respect and the financial rewards that befit the "heros of humanity."[25]

> There is no man in any community more valuable ... than a ... physician. Others may bring personal comforts, wealth and material conveniences, but upon the doctor the people must rely to guard their physical welfare; ... to preserve for young and old life, health and happiness. In mere money the value of his services can never be counted.[25(p33)]

"Mere money," however, is paramount for physicians to determine whether they will even render their holy services. Blatant fostering of physician deification for profit continues today. A physician currently travels throughout the country presenting his lecture entitled "A Course in Miracles." Those willing to "donate" $15.00 per person may attend.[26]

The use of myth and magic gives physicians coercive power. When physicians set themselves up as gods, clients are led to believe that physicians are all-powerful, all-knowing deities.

The use of myth and magic gives physicians coercive power. When physicians set themselves up as gods, clients are led to believe that physicians are all-powerful, all-knowing deities who control by virtue of divinely granted power. A 1935 *Lancet* article illustrates how completely society has been deceived. The author says that physicians are not human at all; on some occasions they are divinity. "We implore (the physician's) presence ... hail his coming with gratitude ... He takes immediate and entire charge of the situation ... he orders us and we obey without question and with trembling eagerness."[27(p800)] The magical qualities fostered by medicine are evident in the author's conclusion that the physician's very presence calms fears, soothes pain and restores hope.

Information Control

Controlling and withholding information can be powerful tools of paternalistic deception. Practitioners of such deception claim benevolence, concern for the deceived. "Humanity fears the unknown so hang a label on his ailment and then he'll endure almost anything. Be explicit about this, even though you may not have the slightest idea what's the matter with him. ... Tell him anything—a man is never frightened of a thing he knows about—or thinks he knows."[27(p801)] The deceived client is dehumanized—amenable to being controlled. By maintaining the client's ignorance the physician is in control.

Ehrenreich and English analyze how deception and control of information have established a model of "expertism" and provided for the economic and social triumph of male medical professionals.

Their study documents that physician control over information makes people dependent upon "medical experts." The basic underlying motivation for this development is the economic factor of selling information to society. Many physicians hoard their knowledge and use it as property to be sold as a commodity. Medicine's goal was not to spread the skills of healing but to concentrate them within the elite group of medicine.[5]

This marketing of information will be ineffective if the client is well informed. Therefore physicians are encouraged (by the AMA, the professional literature, etc.) to maintain control (the paternal role) and to keep clients ignorant (the child role). Physicians are explicitly told how to establish ignorance. They are told to impress on patients that physicians have expert knowledge that is simply unavailable to patients, and to discredit information patients attempt to relate. "Use Latin words with a false concord thrown in; add scientific terms, with a chemical formula or two . . . after that, (the patient) will simply eat out of your hand."[27(p800)]

Corea illustrates that paternalistic deception combines with deception through myth to dehumanize, exploit and control women. She cites the example of women taking DES during pregnancy without their knowledge—a situation that occurred because of physicians' reluctance to give information to women, and the women's own unquestioning faith in their physicians. According to Corea, when some women asked for information about the pills they were told, "The name wouldn't mean anything to you, dear" or "This is a hold-the-baby-in pill."[28(p245)]

Political Pressure

As a political pressure group, the AMA has used various forms of deception. Although the intent has been to bolster profit and prestige,[1,8] the deceptions have been presented to consumers under the guise of various altruistic motives. The most frequent such motive is to save society from communism and socialized medicine.[8] Bok indicates that such deceptive tactics instill fear. Fear then becomes a coercion.[20] In 1944 AMA president Kretschmer illustrated this coercive tactic when he addressed the association membership, discrediting efforts to socialize medicine and calling for the preservation of "the American way of life."[29] The American way of life, in the view of organized medicine, required the physician to be in control of people's minds, feelings and behavior, as well as their pocketbooks. When Kretschmer outlined the strategy to "acquaint" people with the hazards of socialized medicine, he in fact proposed a plan for deception based on misinformation and fear. The fear strategy emphasized that socialized medicine will result in deterioration in the quality of medical care and education, abolition of patients' free choice of physicians and an increase in taxes due to overexpanding bureaucracy.[29]

Politically, organized medicine has inestimable potential. Every day physicians throughout the United States can converse with and possibly convert some two and a half million patients.[8] When the potential for deception in these relationships is considered, the enormity of medicine's power becomes evident.

POLITICAL ABUSE AND EXPLOITATION OF WOMEN

The AMA uses its member physicians to enhance the association's power. It does this by directing the members to deliver public addresses, the texts of which are often furnished by AMA state or national headquarters.[7] The members in turn use their wives to promote medicine's interests by getting them to devote their energy to the work of the medical society via medical auxiliaries. These exploited wives through their activities and behavior indicate their identification with the oppressor—a phenomenon described by Freire.[14] Working through medical society auxiliaries, these women have become commodities to be used by medicine. Bard illustrates the extent that physicians' wives unwittingly accept their commercial status in her writings about her own duties as a physician's wife and about the lives of other wives.[30] Mrs. Maxwell Lick, president of the Pennsylvania Medical Wives Auxiliary, indicates her own oppression and her intention to perpetuate it in a letter to other wives: "This is a busy month for all homes, and as physicians' wives, we have our abundant share of duties. . . . our homes and the medical profession are one and the same." Other wives, she continues, "must be made to realize their responsibilities. . . . This legislative year may prove very important to each physician's home. We cannot afford any type of socialization . . . must give sympathetic support to our profession."[31]

In an article published in a 1944 issue of *JAMA*, Davison illustrated that women physicians are also exploited by medicine—they are objectified and discarded when no longer needed. He suggested how to handle possible overcrowding of the medical profession after World War II: ". . . fill the 20% of each class . . . with students ineligible for military duty (cripples and women) who can treat the civilian population."[32] Medicine's paternalistic deception justified this as "good, for women physicians, being 'expendable' through marriage and retirement after the war, probably will remove approximately 15% from the expected after-war overload."[32]

More than two decades later male physicians continued to use their female counterparts for personal economic gain. In 1966 a medical journal advised physicians: "If your practice could use another M.D.—but only part time—look around for a woman doctor with children. That's the advice of Dr. Seymour I. Kummer, a Connecticut G.P. who employs two M.D.-mothers to do physicals, exams and hospital summaries. A good place to start looking for the ladies: American Medical Women's Association."[33(p187)] In accepting this advice, not only is the male physician relieved of all the so-called "scut" work, but he has the equivalent of a full-time physician without paying for the usual employee benefits (vacations, etc.).

The male medical profession continued to exploit women physicians throughout the 1970s. In 1977 a woman physician illustrated the struggle and final acceptance of her divided life imposed as a result of her sex. In an article published in the official American Academy of Pediatrics newsletter she expounded on the limitations necessary in her practice because she is a woman.[34]

Community Acceptance of Control

The overriding concept of professional control and the social sanction for this control come from the community. The people give the medical profession its power. But the people are deterred from retrieving the power they have bestowed on the medical profession by the deception and myths that surround the profession. Medical deception and myths sedate society to the extent that people become ignorant of what is happening to them. Society remains unaware of their potential power over the medical profession. Consumers can significantly influence medicine once the deceptive practices and medical myths are exposed.

Certain professions are as lulled into mental numbness as society has been. Sociology in particular has idolized medicine and set it up as the "model" of authority without a critical examination of the model's impact on society. Nursing and society continue to adhere to the intolerable situation medicine has created because they are mentally and spiritually bound by the shackles of silence, secrets, lies and ignorance perpetuated throughout history.

The Symbiotic Nurse-Physician Relationship

Historically medicine and nursing have shared a symbiotic relationship in which medicine dominates. As a result of this bond, medicine directly influences nursing's exploitation. This exploitation is based on the concept of conflicting interests: medicine is characteristically disease oriented and derives profit from illness, whereas nursing claims it is health oriented. It is in the area of preventive health care that the conflict between nursing and medicine is most evident. The basic concept of preventive health care denotes health promotion and disease prevention. Medicine profits from keeping humanity sick or making it sick. Therefore the medical profession has a conflict of interest in keeping humanity healthy. A physician writes, "Preventive medicine constantly strives to eradicate that by which it lives."[35(p147)]

Medicine practices paternalistic deception on nurses to lure them into believing that nurses and physicians can work as a

---

Medicine practices paternalistic deception on nurses to lure them into believing that nurses and physicians can work as a team, with the physician as "team captain."

---

team, with the physician as the "team captain." Physicians fear that nurses who are not bound to medicine will realize their own power potential and diminish the power of organized medicine. The objectification of nurses is illustrated in a medical journal's description of the perfect nurse: "She must feel like a girl, act like a lady, think like a man and work like a dog."[36] Ashley proposes that the relationship between medicine and nursing is based on the myth of the holy marriage between nursing and medicine. She explains physicians' assumption that nurses are tied to physicians as legal, subservient partners much like wives are tied to their husbands.[37(p14)] Just as wives are expected to serve their husbands, nurses are expected to serve physicians. Sociologists further this myth by analyzing the physician-patient relationship using a paternalistic (father-child) typology.[38(p323)] It follows that the nurse is the wife/mother in this relationship. As such the nurse takes over the menial chores and performs delegated tasks. Stern reveals his acceptance and promotion of the marriage myth in these words: "Doctors must not divorce themselves from supervising the nursing profession; doctors must not loosen the reins!"[39(p444-446)]

Kissam examines medical delegation in terms of nurse practitioners' "helping out" in rural areas so that physicians may remain in the wealthier cities. He indicates that the political power and economic interests of physicians are well served by maintaining strict controls over the expanded medical delegation that physicians describe as the nurse practitioner's role.[40] A *New England Journal of Medicine* article more clearly shows that "expansion" of nursing's role is actually a tightening of the reins held by physicians, but again this is marked by duplicity. The authors explain that "upgrading the professional nurse" relieves the physician shortage by teaching nurses to use otoscopes and stethoscopes, and collect clinical data. "They are given experi-ence ... within the traditional limits of the physician's overall supervision."[41(p1478)] The physician-author Darley explains how this "upgrading" trains the nurse to fit into the hierarchy of a hospital under a physician's supervision, thereby fostering paternalistic medicine.

REJECTING THE MEDICAL MODEL

In spite of the evidence illustrating nurse exploitation by physicians, nurses seem enamored of the medical model. This acceptance of medicine's paternalism indicates a lack of political sophistication. Nurses have not questioned deeply enough their ties to physicians. Nurses are allowing themselves to be deceived into believing that knowledge of additional medical procedures is expansion. This is medicine's subtle way of reenforcing deceptive ignorance on the part of nurses: paternal medicine's promotion of female mind sedation by discouraging critical questions. Daly suggests that women peel off the layers of mindbindings and false realities to demystify patriarchal lies.[3(p6)] Nurses will then be free to think and create new levels of health for themselves and their clients that are impossible when encumbered with deception. Nurses' most political act will be that of seeing through the deception they have lived with throughout history.

REFERENCES

1. Krause, E. *Power and Illness* (New York: Elsevier 1977).
2. Illich, I. *Medical Nemesis* (New York: Pantheon Books 1976).
3. Daly, M. *Gyn/Ecology: The Metaethics of Radical Feminism* (Boston: Beacon Press 1978) p. 30.
4. Ehrenreich, B. and English, D. *For Her Own Good: 150 Years of the Experts' Advice to Women* (Garden

City, N.Y.: Anchor Press/Doubleday 1978).

5. Ehrenreich, B. and English, D. *Witches, Midwives and Nurses: A History of Women Healers* (New York: The Feminist Press 1973).

6. Stevens, R. *American Medicine and the Public Interest* (New Haven, Conn.: Yale University Press 1972).

7. Lovell, M. "An Historical Study of the Development of the Medical Profession as a Business: Impact on Nursing and Society, 1896-1979," master's thesis, Wright State University, Dayton, Ohio, 1980.

8. Vollmer, H. and Mills, D. *Professionalization* (Englewood Cliffs, N.J.: Prentice-Hall 1966).

9. Harris, R. *A Sacred Trust* (New York: The New American Library 1966).

10. Olson, M. *The Logic of Collective Action: Public Goods and the Theory of Groups* (Cambridge, Mass.: Harvard University Press 1965).

11. Garceau, O. *The Political Life of the American Medical Association* (Cambridge, Mass.: Harvard University Press 1941).

12. Truman, D. B. *The Governmental Process: Political Interests and Public Opinion* 2nd ed. (New York: Alfred A. Knopf 1971) p. 171.

13. *Webster's Third New International Dictionary* Vol. I: A to G (Chicago: Encyclopedia Britannica, William Benton, Publisher 1966).

14. Freire, P. *Pedagogy of the Oppressed* (New York: The Seabury Press 1968).

15. Feldstein, M. "The Medical Economy." *Sci Amer* 229:3 (September 1973) p. 151-159.

16. Rich, A. *On Lies, Secrets, and Silence: Selected Press, 1966-1978* (New York: W. W. Norton & Co. 1979).

17. Gilman, C. P. *The Yellow Wallpaper* (New York: The Feminist Press 1973); reprint of the 1899 edition published by Small, Maynard, Boston.

18. Millett, K. *Sexual Politics* (New York: Doubleday and Co. 1969).

19. Chesler, P. *Women and Madness* (New York: Doubleday and Co. 1972).

20. Bok, S. *Lying: Moral Choice in Public and Private Life* (New York: Vintage Books 1979).

21. Ashley, J. *Hospitals, Paternalism, and the Role of the Nurse* (New York: Teacher's College Press 1976).

22. *Code of Medical Ethics* adapted by the National Medical Convention, Philadelphia, May 1847; and the Medico Chirurgical Society of Cincinnati, March, 1848. *With a Fee Bill* (Cincinnati: J. Ernst).

23. Bressler, B. "When the Magic Runs Out for Doctors." *Psychol Today* 11:2 (July 1977).

24. Helfman, E. *Signs and Symbols around the World* (New York: Lothrop, Lee & Shepard Co. 1967).

25. Taylor, J. J. *The Physician as a Business Man, or, How to Obtain the Best Financial Results in the Practice of Medicine* (Philadelphia: The Medical World 1891).

26. *Jampolski: Seminar & Workshop: A Course in Miracles.* Promotional pamphlet. (Centerville, Ohio: Wholeman Institute 1979).

27. Beith, J. "The Privileged Profession." *Lancet* 2 (October 5, 1935).

28. Corea, G. *The Hidden Malpractice: How American Medicine Treats Women as Patients and Professionals* (New York: William Morrow and Co. 1977).

29. Kretschmer, H. L. "American Medicine and the War." *JAMA* 125:7 (June 17, 1944) p. 461-463.

30. Bard, M. *The Doctor Wears Three Faces* (Philadelphia: J. B. Lippincott Co. 1949).

31. Lick, Mrs. M. "The Woman's Auxiliary." *Penn Med J* 44:3 (December 1940) p. 398-399.

32. Davison, W. "Readjustments of Returning Medical Officers." *JAMA* 124:13 (March 25, 1944) p. 818.

33. "Professional Briefs." *Med Econ* 43:2 (January 1966).

34. Bayes, B. "Mothers and Careers: A Personal Viewpoint." *News & Comments* 28:2 (February 1977).

35. Wolf, G. *The Physician's Business: Practical and Economic Aspects of Medicine* 3rd ed. (Philadelphia: J. B. Lippincott Co. 1944).

36. Pratt, H. "The Doctor's View of the Changing Nurse-Physician Relationship." *J Med Educ* 40:8 (August 1965) p. 767-771.

37. Ashley, J. A. "Nursing Power: Viable, Vital, Visible." *Texas Nurs* (August 1976).

38. Freeman, H., Levine, S. and Reeder, L., eds. *Handbook of Medical Sociology* 2nd ed. (Englewood Cliffs, N.J.: Prentice-Hall 1972).

39. Stern, E. W. "The Responsibility of the Doctor of Medicine in the Training of Nursing Personnel and the Governing of Nursing Care Policy in the Modern Hospital." *Surgery* 46:2 (August 1959) p. 444-446.

40. Kissam, P. C. "Physicians Assistant and Nurse Practitioner Laws: A Study of Health Law Reform." *Univ Kansas Law Review* 24 (Fall 1975) p. 1-65.

41. Darley, W. and Somers, A. R. "Medicine, Money and Manpower—the Challenge to Professional Education." *N Engl J Med* 276:26 (June 29, 1967).

Are Nurses' Mind Sets Compatible with Ethical Practice?

Mila Ann Aroskar, Ed.D., R.N.
Associate Professor
Public Health Nursing
School of Public Health
University of Minnesota
Minneapolis, Minnesota

ETHICAL NURSING practice often seems like a difficult and elusive goal. Why is this? The understanding and implementation of more ethical nursing practice are a challenge and an obligation for nurses as individuals and for the nursing profession collectively. The underlying assumption is that more ethical practice is a "good" to be sought in the delivery of nursing and health care. Understanding and implementation require processes of ethical inquiry, principled thinking, strategies for action and a spirit of compassion for one's self and for others. Nurses have support for more ethical practice in such documents as the ANA Code and ANA Standards for Nursing Practice. Yet one still hears arguments that ethical practice is too risky and requires a certain amount of heroism on the part of nurses.

THE "ETHICAL" IN NURSING PRACTICE

Ethics in nursing has to do with the critical examination of the moral dimensions of decision making at the daily practice level and the policy-making level. The concept of ethical nursing practice indicates practice that is based on and includes critical, reflective thinking about one's duties and obligations as an individual nurse in relation to clients and as a member of a profession fulfilling a social contract. Frequently, there is a lack of clarity as to what counts as the most "right" or "just" judgments, actions and attitudes in delivery of nursing care as a segment of the health care delivery system. A task of nurses and the nursing profession is to determine what is ethical practice in the context of the social contract between hospitals, other employing agencies, physicians and nurses and the larger social contract between a service profession and society. This task is not made easier by the shifting values evident in major social institutions such as families, economics, health, politics and education.

Marilyn Ferguson, author of *The Aquarian Conspiracy*, characterizes these personal and social shifts in society as paradigm shifts. Paradigm shifts have to do with new frameworks, perspectives and ways of thinking about old problems. In health care, changes such as the following are occurring: specialization is giving way to integration and concern for the whole person; emphasis on human values rather than efficiency is gaining; the patient is being viewed as autonomous rather than dependent; and the view of the professional as authority is shifting to one of the professional as therapeutic partner.[1] In these shifts, there are underlying tensions between the value of individual autonomy and the value of the common good in seeking a more just system.

NURSES AND DECISION-MAKING ENVIRONMENTS

Nurses as individual systems interact with other individual systems such as clients or colleagues in the environment. They also interact with larger and more complex social systems such as families and employing agencies which are generally bureaucratic and hierarchical in organization. Each of these systems has its own environments. The environments of nurses and nursing practice include two major dimensions. One dimension relates to the nurse's own internal environment, that is, the individual's own inner world. This world includes a mind set about the systems in which nursing and health care are delivered. The second dimension is the external environment. The external environment includes the mind sets of other individual systems such as providers and patients and the structures of the larger social systems within which these individuals interact.

The internal and external environments of individuals and the larger social systems including their formal and informal policies and norms are interacting and interdependent. They are often the context and source of actual and potential conflict for nurses who seek to achieve a more ethical level of practice.[2,3] See Figure 1 for a way of visualizing the dynamics of environments that impact on ethical practice in nursing.

INTERNAL ENVIRONMENTS AS MIND SETS

Internal as well as external environments affect if and how nurses deal with the

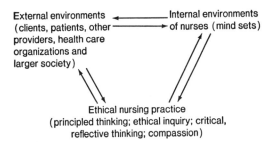

External environments (clients, patients, other providers, health care organizations and larger society) ←——— Internal environments of nurses (mind sets)

Ethical nursing practice
(principled thinking; ethical inquiry; critical, reflective thinking; compassion)

Figure 1. Environments affecting ethical practice.

ethical dimensions of practice. One aspect of the nurse's internal environment is the nurse's mind set or characterization of the health care system. The health care system includes medicine, nursing and other types of services to care for the sick and to promote, restore or maintain health of individuals, groups and communities. Mind sets about health care can be characterized in at least four ways to include:

1. health care as medical cases or scientific projects with the cure of diseases as the single most important object;
2. health care as a commodity in the marketplace;
3. health care as the patient's right to relief from pain or a debilitating condition; and
4. health care as the promotion, maintenance and restoration of health within a cooperative community.

These views are adapted from an article by a philosopher, Lisa Newton.[4] They are used here to represent mind sets of nurses that influence efforts to achieve more ethical practice.

Health care as medical cases

The first mind set—health care as medical cases or scientific projects with the cure of disease as the major goal—may predom-

inate for nurses. It views the hospital or clinic as the "doctor's workshop." The physician may be viewed as the scientist who carries on projects with the hospital as the laboratory. Hospitals or clinics, including administrative activities, exist to facilitate these projects. Patients are the subject matter or case material. Nurses and other health care workers in the system carry on projects subsumed under those of the physician with nursing activities focused on meeting medical goals. Nurses are primarily accountable to physicians for their cases or projects. Medical values dominate the system in the decision-making processes related to patient care, services available and research conducted.

The legitimate focus of nursing activities for nurses who hold this as their predominant mind set about health care is the following of physician orders. The nurse may feel that it is inappropriate to question

---

The legitimate focus of nursing activities for nurses who view health care as medical cases or scientific projects is the following of physician orders.

---

or challenge physicians (still generally men) as the dominant authority figures under this view, even though the nurse may feel uncomfortable about decisions that are made for patients and families by physicians in a primarily paternalistic mode. Other consequences may include feeling blocked or frustrated with few or no options for personal, professional or institutional change. Or, nurses may unquestioningly equate ethical practice with following the wishes and orders of physicians. In some instances, this will be directly antithetical to the view that an appropriate activity of nursing is patient advocacy and to the current ANA Code which views the nurse as a competent professional with specific obligations to clients and society. Note that versions of the code as late as 1950 stated that the nurse's obligation was to carry out physician orders and to protect physicians' reputations. Nurse practice acts also contributed to the view of nurses as subservient to physicians. Efforts to change these practice acts in the past decade have not gone unchallenged.

Consider the power of this view in light of the following findings. Historically, the family was the institutional model for the operation of hospitals. This model still predominates in some hospitals and medical centers. The proper role of women, that is, nurses, was to care for this family and to keep it happy. Nurses were responsible for meeting the needs of all members of the hospital family—from patients to physicians. While nurses were capable of making decisions about patient care in the absence of physicians, they relinquished this role when the physicians returned. Nurses were also to be supportive and loyal to the institution and to preserve its reputation as well as that of the physicians.[5] This view of the appropriate role for nursing is radically different from that of the highly trained and appropriately remunerated professional envisioned by Nightingale more than a century ago.

Findings of a study done in the late 1970s of the moral reasoning of nurses including staff nurses and supervisors in hospitals and public health nursing agencies suggest that most of the participants were at a conventional level of reasoning. Participants at the conventional level stressed obedience to authority and the need for maintaining harmonious relationships with institutions and authority figures "even when patients' rights were being violated."[6] "Blame avoidance" behaviors of nurses are further evidence that they hold a mind set about health care as medical projects as exhibited in statements such as "the doctor ordered it" or "hospital rules require it."

One can still find arguments in the nursing literature in the 1980s for the subordinate role of nurses as functional in the contexts of medicine and hospitals where it is assumed that patients would be placed in jeopardy if health care providers other than physicians were making autonomous judgments about patient care. This assumes that physicians are always on the scene when the need for making clinical decisions does arise. Certainly, this is not a reflection of reality even in many intensive care units to say nothing of emergency rooms and other patient care units. Arguing for the maintenance of the nurse's subordinate role in the hospital environment, the author goes on to say that patients are comfortable with someone in such a role to whom they can ventilate safely. They can ventilate safely because the nurse can do nothing to change the patient's course of treatment. Nurses are seen, according to this author, as having no more control over the environment than patients.[7]

Speculations that nurse practitioners might demonstrate new patterns of behavior in relation to physicians are challenged by a report of in-depth interviews with 28 nurse practitioners. While these nurse practitioners saw themselves as providing a type of care that is currently lacking and desirable in the health care system, they still accommodate to the needs of physicians. They do this by submitting to the limits imposed by the medical profession. Nurse practitioners are legally accountable for their own practice, but the scope of their activities is generally established by physicians or the employing institution. It seems that they accept these restrictions for job security reasons and do so by remaining unobtrusive. Again, the nurse practitioners in this sample saw themselves as having little control over changes necessary to alter the nurse's traditional dependence on the medical community.[8]

The mind set of nursing as subordinate to medicine in health care delivery is still compelling for many nurses in the system. This mind set may well impede efforts to achieve more ethical practice which requires critical, reflective thinking and challenges to the decision-making structure of the present system.

Health care as a commodity

Under the mind set that views health care as a commodity to be sold in the marketplace, health care, that is, nursing and medical care, is offered for sale by hospitals and other health care agencies with the patient as a consumer or customer. The physician is an outside contractor and the nurse is an institutional employee. Under this view, the nurse's primary responsibility is to the administrative hierarchy of the institution. Institutional interests take precedence over the competing interests of traditional professional privi-

leges such as those of the physician. They also take precedence over patient expectations and demands. Examples of this view as it relates more specifically to nursing may be seen in hospitals where packages of nursing services are offered to the patient/consumer or in agencies where competition for clients and the marketing of services become a major focus of nursing activities.

If this is the predominant view of health care held by nursing administrators and by staff, it follows that decisions would be based on a more utilitarian model. Using a utilitarian approach, one attempts to maximize utility or happiness for society and for the greatest number of people. One looks to consequences of alternative choices for the largest group. This approach is directly contradictory to the patient-centered ethic.

The patient-centered ethic is the traditional medical ethic which most nurses and health care providers are imbued with during their professional education. The patient-centered ethic commits nurses to meeting needs of individual patients, which, under this view of health care, often conflicts with the utilitarian goals of the institution. As an employee of the institution, the nurse then undoubtedly opts for primary accountability to the institution rather than to patients thus upholding the goals of the institution. Or, nurses may feel the tremendous conflict which they have not had opportunities to learn to deal with constructively in many education or practice settings. This may be changing as institutions and the profession seek to deal with the stresses of nursing practice in complex social systems. Changes are occurring with development of new staffing patterns such as primary nursing and through such efforts as passage of the ANA resolution on teaching of ethics in continuing education and in basic nursing curriculums.

The point is that nurses who hold the view of health care as predominantly a commodity, whether or not it is consciously recognized, may not question openly what is right or wrong in terms of their own practice as long as it is congruent with institutional goals and policies. This may happen even if they feel personally uncomfortable. It was not too long ago that nurses were exhorted in nursing textbooks to follow the policies of the hospital in order to be ethical. Ethical concerns may not be raised at any system level if the bottom-line ethic in nursing administration is to view health care as a commodity like any other in the marketplace.

This view completely negates the viewpoint that claims there is something special about health care as a service to society. Energies will probably be focused on such issues as competition with other institutions and agencies and the marketing of services rather than the maintenance of standards and the troublesome and difficult ethical issues in delivery of nursing care where issues such as distributive justice constantly intrude. (Distributive justice has to do with who receives the benefits and who bears the burdens of decision making under some concept of need, equality of opportunity, equity or desert.) In reality, institutional interests related to survival are paramount with the current emphasis on cost containment and competition in the delivery of health care

Under the view of health care as the patient's right to relief from pain or a debilitating condition, hospitals exist in society to implement this right for clients who choose to come to these facilities.

services. Yet sensitive nursing administrators and staff are often worried about issues such as justice in their decision making.

Health care as the patient's right to relief from pain

Under the view of health care as the patient's right to relief from pain or a debilitating condition, hospitals and clinics exist in society to implement this right for clients who choose to come to these facilities. The nurse's primary obligation, along with that of other providers, is to meet needs and wants as identified by patients. Patient interests, rather than institutional or medical interests, would dictate what providers' roles would be appropriate in the system.

A major difficulty in implementing this view is that frequently patients identify different needs than those identified by nurses as providers. The patient (or family) might identify his or her need or preference for a private duty nurse while the nurse identifies a higher level of patient independence as more therapeutic. Or a new teenage mother's view of her needs may differ radically from that of the public health nurse who may see the mother's ideas as putting her infant in jeopardy. Under this view, the needs identified by the client based on his or her values would be decisive. This view of needs also raises the specter of health care delivery attempting to deal with a bottomless pit of identified needs or demands.

Some nurses have expressed opinions that this is a more desirable model from their points of view based on the promotion of a patient advocate role for nurses and meeting of patient needs as a primary goal of nursing care. However, this view logically puts the nurse then in the position of acting as an instrument to carry out what the patient wishes with patient values predominating. One wonders what happens to the integrity of nurses as persons and professionals under this view if it is accepted unquestioningly as ethical nursing practice.

Consumer movements, the Patients' Bill of Rights and some malpractice suits seem to point in the direction of more consumer control of the health care system. This model assumes that patients know what they need and how to use the system to satisfy their identified needs and wants related to health care. Educational efforts are being carried out by lawyers, physicians, nurses and others to assure more sophisticated consumers of health care.[9]

The above three views of the health care system make nurses primarily means to the ends of others. Nurses may be used by institutional administrators, physicians, researchers and patients to achieve goals based on values determined by individuals and groups other than nurses and the nursing community. These views, which may be held consciously or unconsciously by nurses as particular mind sets, have consequences for nurses as individuals and

for the profession. Consequences may include patient care and damage to the nurses' personal and professional integrity. These mind sets may play a major role in the failure to develop more ethical nursing practice even though formal documents exist in support of more ethical practice. This is not to say that ethical practice is, or ever will be, easy.

These mind sets conflict directly or indirectly with the ANA Code which speaks to a broader vision of nursing's duties and obligations in society, with standards of practice developed by the nursing community, and with the development of nursing theories. These and other elements have influenced current nursing practice acts which point to a different view of nursing care within the health care delivery system in terms of responsibility and accountability. In this fourth view, nurses are not instruments of others such as institutions, other providers or patients.

One other possible implication of the above views (perhaps of even more serious import) is that nurses use other nurses to meet institutional, medical or client goals rather than questioning the appropriateness of these mind sets for nurses and nursing.

Health care as promotion of well-being in a cooperative community

According to the view of health care as the promotion, maintenance and restoration of client well-being in a cooperative community, all participants' values are taken into account in decision-making processes at various system levels such as one-to-one interactions and policy making. This is a process that respects the values of the individuals involved in or affected by the decisions. The client is still the focus of care delivery, but the process implies that all participants are individually respected for their contribution to the goal of maximizing the individual's optimum level of health rather than simply means to the ends of others. Both providers and clients have rights and responsibilities under this view of health care delivery.

This view is not a panacea for all the problems in the system. For example, it could lead to a "blame-the-victim" syndrome in which clients would be considered responsible for their own conditions even though causes of the condition have not been identified (such as some types of cancer or alcoholism). This view could and does result in the asking of different questions and raises different concerns for nurses and others in regard to what constitutes more ethical nursing practice. Should, for example, nurses be responsible and accountable in the system for ensuring that clients have input into decisions affecting their futures?

IMPLICATIONS OF MIND SETS FOR ETHICAL PRACTICE

Each of the views discussed has implications for the ways in which nurses do, or do not, identify ethical issues and dilemmas in their practice. Each represents a mind set that has the potential for different nursing judgments, attitudes and actions in relation to how individual nurses and groups of nurses deal with ethical concerns and how they are interpreted. The added significance of these mind sets is that they are held not solely by nurses but also by the people with whom nurses interact such as other health providers, administrators, patients and families. These mind sets are then part of the nurse's internal *and* external environments.

Under the first three views of health care, one could say that the nurse whose practice is congruent with the goals of the employing institution, the medical community or clients is engaging in what could be considered to be at least morally correct if not ethical practice. Only the last view focuses on nurses as more individually and professionally responsible and accountable at a higher level than the legal minimum requirements of the other views. Under this last view, no persons are considered simply as means to the ends of others. Principled thinking, related to respect for individuals, would suggest that all individuals involved as providers and recipients of health care would be required to scrutinize their judgments, attitudes and actions in light of their impact on others' autonomy and values.

This is not meant to suggest that the first three views are necessarily immoral. Rather they are limited in terms of their requirements for the most fully ethical practice of nursing, if one views ethical practice on a continuum from less ethical to more ethical and considers requirements such as principled thinking, ethical inquiry and critical, reflective thinking. Thus the last view or "newer" view proposes a new paradigm for thinking about health care in which respect for all the individuals involved in or affected by major decisions to be made points to a different process and structure for the making of those decisions. The last view is implied in many current nursing documents and in professional and lay literature.

STRATEGIES AND SUPPORTS FOR NURSES WHO SEEK MORE ETHICAL PRACTICE

First, and perhaps most difficult, the acquisition of a new mind set requires that one acknowledge and give up the other mind sets where nurses are primarily means to the ends of others. This requires a change in one's own inner world, the internal environment. While it is evident that nursing and health care literature, significant nursing documents and many nurses in service, education and research are working to bring this new mind set to bear on delivery of care, it is also evident that many are comfortable with the old paradigms for decision making. While nurses may rail against the old paradigms as demeaning, they may also use them "to blame" others for what happens or does not happen in nursing care as long as nurses meet their legal responsibilities in practice. Reality is that legal responsibility establishes a bare minimum for practice whereas professional practice implies a higher order of obligations as promulgated by the profession through establishment of a code of ethics, standards of practice, educational requirements for entry into practice, and development of certification processes.

The other side of the coin is society's expectations of nursing. If society's expectations are that nurses simply follow physician orders and provide a safe sounding board, then some of the concerns raised here around a different paradigm or mind set for delivery of nursing and health care are moot. Evidence suggests other possibilities. Some nurses, physicians and consumers are concerned about how health care delivery and decision making are structured at present and how they should be structured in a more humane manner. In addition, alternative modes of health care delivery are being mandated by third party payers such as government and are developing from needs of consumers such as self-help groups that use professionals as consultants or in an educational capacity.

Our society and profession seem to value action and "busyness" per se. On the other hand, existing conditions of practice in many settings allow for little else. When do nurses on a busy hospital unit, in a crowded nursing home or in a community nursing agency with a heavy caseload have an opportunity to think through together the nursing care issues and challenges with which they are confronted at conscious or nonconscious levels?

Many of these issues and concerns have repercussions in judgments, actions and attitudes toward practice. Many have ethical dimensions related to distributive justice in the sense of the most "right" or "just" distribution of scarce nursing resources—a valuable and necessary social resource both locally and nationally. Or there are questions and worries about how decisions are made by and for patients or clients. One could argue that nursing administrators have an obligation to plan with their staff for staffing patterns that allow for such opportunities perhaps in an

It is appalling to discover how frequently nurses are unaware that they are involved in situations requiring consideration of ethical elements.

ethical rounds format where the purpose is to discuss the ethical dimensions of a patient care situation or a program change. It is appalling to discover how frequently nurses are unaware that they are involved in situations requiring consideration of ethical elements. An example is a nursing supervisor in a nursing home who said that she had no ethical dilemmas, yet there were elderly patients who were comatose and on respirators, and who were transported for renal dialysis. Nurses followed established medical protocols.

Hospital nursing administrators and staff nurses could look for support for the newer paradigm in the Nursing Services Section of the *JCAH Accreditation Manual for Hospitals* (1982 edition). Standards have been developed based on the principle that the nursing department "takes all reasonable steps to provide the optimal achievable quality of nursing care and to maintain the optimal professional conduct and practices of its members."[10] Interpretations of standards include the requirement that a sufficient number of qualified RNs are available to give patients care that requires the judgment and specialized skills of RNs to achieve quality nursing care and a safe patient environment. Nursing care plans are individualized with goals set mutually with the patient and/or family whenever this is possible. While these standards are to be implemented consistent with the medical plan of care, they denote a more interdependent process of nursing responsibility and accountability that is more consistent with the view of a cooperative community of health care delivery.

The ANA document, *Nursing: A Social Policy Statement* (1980), is a formulation of nursing's social responsibility and is also more congruent with the cooperative community view of health care delivery. One might well ask where the professional and public arenas exist for discussion of this and other nursing documents which articulate nursing leaders' views of the profession. Basic consciousness-raising endeavors are needed within the profession and with other providers and the public that nursing serves.

Muyskens, a philosopher, argues that the notion of collective responsibility in nursing is "a weapon" to be used in seeking more ethical nursing practice by individuals and the profession through the development of organizational mechanisms for implementation of the ANA Code. While these mechanisms do exist in the profession nationally and in the professional nursing organizations in many states, they do not exist in all states or in all nursing service organizations. On the other hand, even if the mechanisms do exist, individuals may not know about them in order to use them.

Muyskens argues that while individuals may do all that is required of them, their responsibilities are still greater than someone who is not a member of the profession to work toward upgrading the group's conduct when it is below the professional standards that can reasonably be expected of that group.[11] Can the nursing profession claim that its standards are met in all practice settings? Or do the standards need to be changed? A critical example would be unsafe patient environments by virtue of a lack of adequate nursing staff in terms of numbers and necessary expertise.

The notion of invoking collective responsibility requires sensitive individuals within (or outside?) a profession who can articulate their concerns based on principles of "rightness" and the existence of a compatible mind set. Nurses who hold mind sets emphasizing health care as a commodity where institutional interests take precedence over other interests, health care as physician projects, or health care as implementation of patient rights where nurses are essentially means to the ends of others, may be paying a high price in terms of personal and professional integrity. There is conceivably a cost to the health care system in terms of their potential contributions as responsible professionals.

There is also a cost to the profession in terms of lack of progress on the journey toward more ethical nursing practice.

While there are no panaceas, there are assessment efforts that could be made in the nurse's inner world and in the nursing profession to deal as responsibly and effectively as possible with efforts to achieve more ethical nursing practice if individuals and the profession so determine. Have you identified your own current mind set on nursing within the health care delivery system? Perhaps this is a necessary step toward more ethical practice in nursing in complex social systems.

REFERENCES

1. Ferguson, M. *The Aquarian Conspiracy* (Los Angeles: J.P. Tarcher 1980) p. 246-248.
2. Davis, A.J. and Aroskar, M.A. *Ethical Dilemmas and Nursing Practice* (New York: Appleton-Century-Crofts 1978) p. 31-44.
3. Murphy, C.P. "The Moral Situation in Nursing" in Bandman, E.L. and Bandman, B., eds. *Bioethics and Human Rights* (Boston: Little, Brown 1978) p. 313-320.
4. Newton, L.H. "To Whom Is the Nurse Accountable? A Philosophical Perspective." *Connecticut Medicine* 43:10 (1979) p. 7-9.
5. Ashley, J.A. *Hospitals, Paternalism, and the Role of the Nurse* (New York: Teachers College Press 1976) p. 17.
6. Murphy. "The Moral Situation in Nursing." p. 315.
7. Newton, L.H. "In Defense of the Traditional Nurse." *Nursing Outlook* 29:6 (1981) p. 348-354.
8. Simmons, R.S. and Rosenthal, J. "The Women's Movement and the Nurse Practitioner's Sense of Role." *Nursing Outlook* 29:6 (1981) p. 371-375.
9. Gots, R. and Kaufman, A. *The People's Hospital Book* (New York: Avon Books 1981).
10. Joint Commission on Accreditation of Hospitals. *Accreditation Manual for Hospitals* 1982 ed. (Chicago: JCAH 1982) p. 115.
11. Muyskens, J.L. "Collective Responsibility and the Nursing Profession" in Mappes, T.A. and Zembaty, J.S., eds. *Biomedical Ethics* (New York: McGraw-Hill 1981) p. 102-108.

Solving Ethical Dilemmas in Nursing Practice

Margot Joan Fromer, M.Ed., R.N.
Freelance Writer and
Nursing Consultant
Washington, D.C.

ALL NURSES WHO work with clients face ethical dilemmas every day, sometimes several times a day, and most know that they *ought* to do or say something, to take a stand. Most of the time, however, they do nothing. They continue about their work, albeit with a vague sense of uneasiness, until the next dilemma occurs and the process repeats itself. If the nurse is an ethically sensitive person, sufficient experiences of this sort may create an impression of helplessness and of being powerless to do the correct thing in a given situation.

ETHICAL THEORIES

Before one can attempt to solve ethical dilemmas, it is essential to understand the basis of ethical theory from which one is operating. Although most nurses do not give much conscious thought to having adopted a particular ethical theory on which to base one's professional and non-professional moral decisions, they should be aware that there are two prevalent ethical theories that guide decision making: utilitarianism and deontology.

These theories, and the principles based on them, are extremely complex and have shades and nuances of meaning that make them fascinating to consider. The danger in attempting to describe them briefly is that they may be reduced to mere catch phrases and thus seem to lose some of their importance as theories and principles by which people live. Accordingly, the reader is strongly encouraged to do further study on the subject.

Utilitarianism has often been characterized by the phrase, "the greatest good for the greatest number." This is an oversimplification of the theories found mainly in the writings of Bentham and Mill.[1,2] Utilitarianism holds that an action is morally correct if its consequences produce the greatest amount of happiness for the greatest number of people, including the actor. Note that moral decisions are based solely on the consequences of actions, not on the inherent rightness or wrongness of the actions themselves.

Utilitarianism has frequently been the victim of "bad press" because it is mistakenly associated with only *physical* pleasure and happiness and thus takes on a rather hedonistic cast. Mill, however, countered this objection by stating that intellectual pleasure is a worthier goal than physical pleasure and thus counts for more happiness. Another drawback is that extremely reprehensible actions can be condoned by appealing to utilitarianism. Minority views can be ignored, for instance, because the "greatest-happiness" principle discounts those who fall outside the "greatest number."

Deontology holds that there are features of an act that make it right or wrong regardless of the consequences. An act can be wrong in itself, even if it results in increased happiness. Characteristics that contribute to the rightness or wrongness of an act are truth telling, promise keeping, justice, beneficence, and the like. Deontologic theories are either monistic or pluralistic.

The most widely known proponent of monistic deontology is Kant who formulated the Categorical Imperative—a universally applicable maxim by which all other maxims of action can be tested.[3] Monistic deontology tends to be difficult to apply to modern life, however, and most modern deontologists, such as Ross and Rawls, hold a pluralistic view and acknowledge that several principles can be simultaneously applied to a conflict.[4-6] These principles can be assigned priority, depending

---

Each ethical conflict one faces may call for application of different principles.

---

on the views of the particular problem solver. Each ethical conflict one faces may call for application of different principles, and one is frequently confronted with the dilemma of having to sacrifice some principles in favor of others, depending on the situation.

ETHICAL PRINCIPLES

The four most important principles that pluralistic deontologists tend to consider are autonomy, nonmaleficence, beneficence and justice. These principles are extremely complex and are subject to widely varying interpretation.

Autonomy is the principle discussed most often and thus is the one most familiar to nurses. It is also the principle most ignored when health care is delivered. Autonomy is personal liberty of action and implies independence, self-reliance, freedom of choice and the ability to make decisions. A prisoner may make a decision to go outdoors for an evening stroll, but he does not have the liberty to act on that choice; therefore, he is not autonomous. The point is that autonomy cannot exist in a vacuum; it must be acknowledged and respected by others.

Mill argues that the only permissible reason to remove a person's social or personal autonomy is to prevent harm to *others*. Autonomy cannot be exercised if an individual is living within a social structure in which his or her autonomy is not respected. If a hospitalized person decides not to take a medication, and his care givers somehow coerce him to take it, he does not have autonomy. It can be seen, then, that autonomy may be defined as personal liberty of action, but that it cannot be exercised without the agreement or consent of those controlling the individual's immediate and distant social environment.

Nonmaleficence means the duty to do no harm and is generally considered to be the foundation on which health care delivery rests. It is mentioned prominently in the Hippocratic Oath and forms the basis for most medical and nursing codes of ethics.

On the face of it, it seems relatively easy to understand that health professionals are obligated not to harm clients; in practice, however, nonmaleficence is more complex than it appears. The concept of harm can be defined in a number of ways and includes deliberate harm, risk of harm and harm that occurs during the performance of beneficial actions. Intentional harm is always impermissible, risk of harm is not so clear-cut. One is subject to the risk of death or serious harm during many kinds of surgery and other forms of diagnostic and therapeutic treatments for the purpose of achieving the ultimate benefit of improved health. A conflict exists as to what degree of risk is morally permissible.

Beneficence also seems quite matter-of-fact; it means the doing or active promotion of good, and encompasses all direct and indirect actions. In the health professions, beneficence is usually taken to mean a duty or obligation to confer health benefits on clients. Beauchamp and Childress emphasize that beneficence requires not only a positive provision of benefits, but also a balancing of benefits and harms.[7] In other words, we are obligated as health professionals to produce and provide good, but not if the provision of that good also produces an equal or greater harm.

Therein lies the difficulty. It is almost impossible to ensure benefit without risking harm; as technology increases in complexity, so do the ethical dilemmas. Most people believe that nonmaleficence is a higher principle than beneficence and should take precedence over it. But health professionals also feel a moral obligation to promote good and therefore frequently find themselves locked in ethical conflict.

Justice is the most complex and difficult principle to apply to nursing care. There are many concepts and definitions of justice; for example, it is frequently explained in terms of fairness. In these terms, it is thought that justice is served when an individual receives his or her "just deserts," or what is owed him or her by another individual or by society. Justice almost always involves rights or claims that must be balanced and weighed against each other.

In health care one must frequently use the principle of justice to guide decisions about how to allocate scarce resources. This is true in a large societal context (Who will receive the artificial kidney? How much should be spent on arthritis versus cancer research?). It is also true in the day-to-day practice of individual nurses. For example, when one professional nurse is alone on a unit with 20 or 30 clients, all demanding attention, the nurse must at times rely on a sense of justice in deciding whose needs to attend to first. Which of two people in pain is the more deserving of immediate administration of a narcotic, and who can or should wait a few minutes? The nurse may not realize, when rushing from client to client, that she is facing ethical dilemmas and that if she understood the principles of justice, she might not feel so emotionally torn and unsure of herself while trying to make these decisions. If she could stop and decide that the fairest course of action is based on the situation she faces, her decision making would be more likely to be based on *principle* rather than emotion. In the case of the two clients in pain, the nurse must choose whom to medicate first, and that choice must be made on the basis of the facts at hand, not personal preference or other considerations.

GWEN'S DILEMMA

The following case illustrates how these principles can be applied to the practice of nursing.

Gwen has been a hospital staff nurse for a good many years and had seen thousands of clients come and go. She has forgotten about most of them, but a few have stayed in her mind for one reason or another. When Bonnie was admitted, Gwen recognized her instantly even though ten years had intervened since her last visit. A decade before, when Bonnie was 15, she had been admitted for a therapeutic abortion which her mother had requested and the physician had agreed to perform (this was prior to the 1973 Supreme Court decision [*Roe v. Wade*, 410 U.S. 113] that granted women the right to abortion in the first two trimesters).[8] Bonnie wanted to bear the child, but both her mother and the physician insisted that she was "too young" and that she would "soon forget about it."

Gwen remembered the case so well not only because it was unusual but also because, although Bonnie was unhappy and crying a good deal of the time, she appeared to be an extraordinarily mature adolescent who seemed certain that she did not want an abortion. She had appealed to Gwen for help in trying to convince her mother to let her have the baby. But Gwen, although sympathetic, was busy with her other clients, the mother and physician were very persuasive, and Bonnie *was* only 15 and in an extremely vulnerable position. So the abortion was performed, Bonnie was discharged the following day, sullen but not overtly depressed, and Gwen, aside from a twinge of guilt whenever she thought about the incident, put it mostly out of her mind.

Now Bonnie was admitted again, this time for a diagnostic evaluation for infertility. When Gwen admitted her, she noticed a glint of recognition on Bonnie's face, but it was not until the next day that Bonnie fully remembered Gwen. The two had a long talk, during which Bonnie said that she had been married for four years and had been unable to conceive. She had not told her husband or her current physician about the abortion, and her mother wholeheartedly agreed with the decision to keep silent. She begged Gwen not to reveal what had happened ten years before.

There are four major dilemmas here that confront both Gwen and Bonnie:

1. Bonnie is withholding important information from her husband and physician. Could this be classed as lying or another form of deceit, and is she morally obligated to reveal that she had had an abortion ten years ago?
2. Gwen now has a piece of information that could significantly affect Bonnie's diagnosis. Is she obligated to reveal it, or may she assure Bonnie of confidentiality?
3. To whom does Gwen owe greater professional loyalty, to Bonnie or to the physician *in this instance?*
4. If Gwen agrees not to tell what she

Gwen has a piece of information that could significantly affect Bonnie's diagnosis. Is she obligated to reveal it, or may she assure Bonnie of her confidentiality?

---

knows, can she be held partially liable for an erroneous diagnosis, and could she be legally culpable?

These questions can all be answered, not to everyone's satisfaction, of course, by using the principles discussed above and by operating from a theoretical base. However, solving the dilemma *in theory* is one thing; the actual practice of nursing and living with whatever decision is made is something else.

The case in theory involves the conflict of loyalty that nurses often experience when they are "pulled" from physician to client and back again. It also is about confidentiality and truth-telling (the first dilemma), two concepts that lead to many similar dilemmas.

Bok defines a lie as an intentionally deceptive message that is stated verbally or in writing;[9] deceit is a much wider-ranging phenomenon which also includes both the indirect attempt to lead people into believing falsehoods and the omission of information that they ought to have. Obviously, Bonnie is deceiving her husband and physician although perhaps not actually lying to them. The fact of her abortion is information that *belongs* to her, and a case can be made both for and against her moral obligation to provide the physician with the information. An abortion a decade before would have little to do with the husband or with his present relationship with Bonnie. However, if Bonnie's infertility could be proved to be causally connected to the abortion, then her obligation to her husband vis à vis the information might change. The nurse's role in this particular aspect of the total dilemma seems more interpersonal than ethical. She might help Bonnie to look at *both* the ethical and psychological ramifications inherent in choosing whether or not to reveal her past, but she must *not* diminish the client's autonomy in this matter, either by telling her what to do or by approving or disapproving of her eventual choice.

The second dilemma is perhaps the most perplexing and is inextricably intertwined with the third. It is true that the information about the abortion belongs to Bonnie, but Gwen knows it also; thus she holds "part ownership." Knowing that Bonnie had been able to become pregnant in the past would certainly alter the physician's diagnostic evaluation, and it may or may not help solve the problem of why she is unable to conceive now. A physician surely has a right to all pertinent data to make an accurate diagnosis, and Bonnie, by her voluntary consent to the diagnostic work-up, has indicated that she too wishes a diagnosis so she can become pregnant; thus she *ought* to want to provide the information. Gwen probably should try to convince Bonnie to voluntarily help herself by being totally candid with the physician. However, if Bonnie still wishes to remain silent, Gwen will have to make a decision.

Almost equally good cases can be made both for and against Gwen's revealing the information, but this ethical decision is perhaps most difficult on a personal level. Either way Gwen decides to resolve the conflict can result in guilt feelings which must be consciously confronted. The most effective way to deal with the personal conflicts produced by this and other ethical dilemmas is to use ethical principles to solve them in the first place. This means using the principles described above (and others if applicable) to apply to situations in which ethical conflicts arise. Nurses should become as used to doing this as they are to applying the principles of physics, biochemistry, psychology and the like to solve other nursing problems. If principles are applied deliberately and consistently, fewer mistakes will be made and less harm will be done to clients and colleagues.

The fourth dilemma is a purely legal matter, and there are two special aspects of which the nurse should be aware. First, many, if not all, professional nursing actions can have legal ramifications. This fact should not prevent nurses from doing the ethically correct thing, but nurses should keep in mind that they may eventually have to justify their actions in court. Second, legally permissible behavior may not necessarily be morally correct, and vice versa. We can all think of many examples of actions that are morally blameworthy but for which we are not legally liable (lying, for example, unless it is done in court under oath) and examples of laws that are immoral. Thus, in making her decision, Gwen must understand not only that legality and morality are not necessarily the same, but also that the ability to adequately justify an action morally may have no legal bearing.

NURSING EDUCATION AND NURSING DILEMMAS

The real tragedy with regard to ethical dilemmas in nursing practice is not that nurses do not recognize that such dilemmas exist; rather it is their lack of preparation to solve these dilemmas using ethical principles. Many see this as the fault of nursing education, which tends to minimize the importance of the humanities in general and moral philosophy in particular. The "hard" sciences in baccalaureate education have received increasingly strong emphasis in the past decade or so. Many believe this to be a mistake because they do not see nurses as scientists, but rather as humanists with a scientific base of knowledge. With a few exceptions, nurses do not care for clients *qua* physiologic beings. They care for clients *qua* human beings. Knowledge of microbiology, anatomy and

physiology, although surely important for nurses, should not obliterate the necessity for studying moral philosophy and the other humanities. It is the study of the humanities that will tend to provide the foundation for dealing with clients as they present themselves to nurses—as whole human beings. Until students seriously study the humanistic aspect of nursing practice, the profession as a whole will remain handicapped when confronted with ethical dilemmas.

REFERENCES

1. Bentham, J. *An Introduction to the Principles of Morals and Legislation* (New York: Hafner Publishing Co. 1948).
2. Mill, J.S. *Utilitarianism, On Liberty, and Essay on Jeremy Bentham.* Warnock, M., ed. (Cleveland: World Publishing 1962).
3. Kant, I. *Groundwork of the Metaphysic of Morals.* Translated by H.J. Paton (New York: Harper and Row 1964).
4. Ross, W.D. *The Right and the Good* (Oxford: Clarendon Press 1930).
5. Ross, W.D. *The Foundations of Ethics* (Oxford: Clarendon Press 1939).
6. Rawls, J.A. *A Theory of Justice* (Cambridge: Harvard University Press 1971).
7. Beauchamp, T.L. and Childress, J.F. *Principles of Biomedical Ethics* (New York: Oxford University Press 1979).
8. *Roe v. Wade*, 410 U.S. 113, 35 L. Ed. 2d 147, 93 S Ct. 705 (1973).
9. Bok, S. *Lying: Moral Choice in Public and Private Life* (New York: Random House 1978).

Authenticity: Fabric of Ethical Nursing Practice

M. Janice Nelson, Ed.D., R.N.
Associate Administrator for Nursing
State University Hospital
Upstate Medical Center
Syracuse, New York

"The willingness to enter with a patient that predicament which he cannot face alone is an expression of moral responsibility; the quality of the moral commitment is a measure of the nurse's excellence."

—Myra E. Levine[1]

AUTHENTICITY—AN EXISTENTIAL THEME

ETHICS, as traditionally presented, embodies certain principles of human behavior which serve as guidelines in the determination of right and wrong. The term *ethical behavior* denotes a level of personal integrity—a certain uprightness of character, honesty in one's choices of action. *Unethical behavior* reflects a moral departure from the right or the good; it is behavior that is, in essence, dishonest, and may, in some instances, be considered evil.

Interwoven throughout the ethical fabric—the rightness or wrongness of human acts—is the notion of *authenticity,* or, from an existential vantage point, the authentic versus the inauthentic life. For purposes of clarification, in everyday language we refer to something being authentic or genuine, such as an antique. In this same vein, the existential notion of living an authentic life essentially means that we are true to ourselves—that we are, in a sense, real or genuine.

Kierkegaard, Sartre, Camus, Marcel and Buber believe that living an authentic life involves committing ourselves to defining our own lives in light of our talents and abilities, taking responsibility for ourselves, being willing to answer for our choices and involving ourselves with all that life has to offer. In addition authenticity denotes truthfulness, individuality and breaking

---

Authenticity involves a certain level of maturity and self-determination, and a willingness to accept personal accountability.

---

with the habitual. It means refusing to be "one of the crowd," being a risk taker and being willing to put oneself on the line. It means acting on a value system we believe in without being willing to compromise those values in order to be with the "in" group. Authenticity also means that each of us, as individuals or "single ones," though part of a larger society, must name our own meanings, and attempt to develop a sense of self-consciousness as to how we intend our world. Authenticity, then, involves a certain level of maturity and self-determination, and a willingness to accept accountability.

The existentialists will admit, however, that there are varying degrees of authenticity, and authenticity may, in fact, be difficult to discern. Often the inauthentic person may be viewed by a neighbor as a "nice" person. This person follows social norms, is a good neighbor, gets along well with people and meets financial obligations. Closer scrutiny, however, reveals that there is a type of distancing between this person and the world; that is, the person lacks personal involvement, fails to take a political stand for fear of recrimination, or is untouched by important human and social events such as the plight of the Vietnamese boat people or the recent hostage situation in Iran. In Marcel's words:

Each of us becomes the center of a sort of mental space arranged in concentric zones of decreasing interest and participation. It is as though each of us secreted a kind of shell which gradually hardened and imprisoned him; and this sclerosis is bound up with the hardening of the categories in accordance with which we conceive and evaluate the world.[2]

A fascinating essay by Sartre entitled *Portrait of the AntiSemite* presents the concept of authentic versus inauthentic life with great clarity.[3] The crucial message embodied in the essay focuses on fear of taking responsibility for one's choices. The antiSemite addressed in the essay is a person who, as Sartre would posit, "lives in bad faith." Although portrayed as a man, the antiSemitic person could be any one of us. The antiSemite is the person who is self-righteous and who fears standing alone, taking responsibility or challenging social mores. Walled in by his prejudices, the antiSemite reflects a man of the crowd who never comes in contact with his inner-self; he lives in a world of social conformity. As Sartre put it: "Authentic liberty recognizes its responsibilities, while the antiSemitic liberty comes from the fact that he flees all responsibility."[4]

Thus, in the extreme, if any of us were that inauthentic person we would care about no one but ourselves; we would be immobilized by our fears; and while we may never admit to being unfeeling, we would never put ourselves in question much less challenge our own existence. We would live comfortably in a world of immunity, insensitivity and unawareness. The problems of the world would not be ours.

Authenticity, on the other hand, lies in acting on one's freedom in terms of self-determination, while concomitantly taking care not to infringe on the rights or freedom of others. Authenticity involves making responsible choices, and being willing to answer for the consequences.

In these times of sophisticated medical procedures and technology, the nurse as well as the patient can easily get caught up, if not lost, in the mechanical menagerie. Now more than ever before the nurse is called upon to assist in decisions regarding patient care that are clearly ethical in nature. Thus, it behooves us to concentrate on how the notion of authenticity relates to nursing practice.

PROFILE OF THE AUTHENTIC NURSE

Individuality

Nursing is a clinical service. Throughout our basic educational preparation, the principal area of focus was on learning basic nursing theory, integrating content from other disciplines such as psychology and sociology, and translating as well as integrating these theories and content into clinical nursing practice. Upon completion of the program, it was not unusual for us to present ourselves to the world of work with stars in our eyes—eager to be of service and equally eager to make a positive contribution to the delivery of nursing care.

Often, the transition from student to professional nurse can be a traumatic experience. Many of us find ourselves enveloped in a highly technologic, automated, bureaucratic system for which we may not be prepared. We may become increasingly aware that the individual can become more and more powerless with respect to the system, and we may find ourselves resisting submergence and a loss of personal identity.

What becomes of essence, then, is how we as nurses, as persons, choose to respond to this environment; how we choose to define ourselves and name our own meanings in a system where things are already named, where tradition, routines and habitual practices prevail. Our authenticity lies in keeping in touch with ourselves as persons, in adhering to a personal value system and having the courage to resist peer pressure for mediocre practice should such pressure exist. This does not mean that we will not aspire to a certain "group belongingness" or participate in team effort—these are essential to personal and professional survival. What it does mean is that we do not succumb to loss of personal identity or abdicate personal responsibility and accountability for our actions. It also means that we guard against becoming immune and insensitive to or alienated from sickness, pain, suffering and death which may be a daily occurrence in our world of work.

An authentic nurse, then, is one who is willing to take the risk of being an individual, one who makes responsible decisions and is willing to answer for them. An example of such a nurse is Christine Smith who exposed information on the high incidence of infant morbidity and maternal infection in a hospital where she worked. After repeated attempts to intervene in an untenable situation, Smith resigned in order to retain her principles. She concluded by saying that nurses, "have a responsibility to know what we need to know to practice, ... [and] also a responsibility to act as advocates for those who cannot speak for themselves. As professionals, we carry a commitment and responsibility to all the people in the community in which we practice."[5]

Not everyone can afford to resign. It is vital, however, that we are *aware;* that we, like Smith, examine all available options before determining a course of action. We owe this to ourselves.

Intersubjectivity

The thrust of existential thought lies in the realm of *being;* that is, that as individuals we spend our lives striving toward full personhood, self-realization and self-actualization. What is involved here is the willingness to act on one's existential freedom and choose to commit oneself to this lifelong endeavor. This process is never finished; we never reach that truly perfect state of being, but once the commitment is made, there is no turning back; we must continue the struggle. Of course, this type of commitment—to live our lives as fully as we can—involves risk, because we can

never really know what the outcome will be; but Marcel says, it is this very notion of risk that gives weight to the commitment.[6]

In conjunction with this, existentialists believe that no one lives out his or her life in isolation—there are always "others." For Buber and Marcel in particular, one's relationship with others has everything to do with one's relationship with the self. We must recognize others as other beings—beings who struggle, love and suffer the same as we do. Marcel asserts: "The more my existence takes on the character of including others, the narrower becomes the gap which separates it from being; the more, in other words, I am."[7]

This phenomenon becomes the crux of the matter when one speaks of authenticity in nursing practice. Sartre's antiSemite betrayed himself while betraying others. While Sartre never seemed to resolve the question of interpersonal relationships (intersubjectivity), he did assert that "choosing for oneself, one is, if consistent, choosing for others as well."[8] Without a doubt, intersubjectivity is at the heart of the ethical question and bears numerous implications for the nurse.

For example, as nurses, we are often faced with ethical situations involving nursing care relating to abortion, disconnecting of life-support systems, issues of informed consent and procedures of behavior modification. Additionally, persons suffering from debilitating diseases, limb dismemberment, radical surgeries, mental illness and the like often have their freedom (physical and mental) severely limited. Given these and other circumstances, those of us who are striving to be authentic will examine the options available in a given situation, act responsibly in the best interest of the patient and be accountable for the action. Moreover, in order to get in touch with the patient, we will mentally put ourselves in the patient's place and attempt to understand the patients' world. The more we can open ourselves to sharing a common situation (inasmuch as it can be shared) with the patient, the more we will be able to relate to this person. The more we can do this, the more authentic we become.

If we are less than authentic, on the other hand, we will more readily adhere to "routine" procedure. We will blindly follow physicians' prescriptions relating to patient care, with little or no concern for the patient's well-being. Or we may relegate the patient to the realm of *it*—some *thing* to be worked on, manipulated and used. In this situation we can become vulnerable to chronic immunity, to keeping a distance between ourselves and patients and to merely "lending" ourselves to our clients— giving nothing and receiving nothing.

The heart of the matter is the identification of a personal value system, how we

---

Not everyone is capable of the same degree of authenticity, but it behooves each of us to strive for the highest degree possible.

---

regard ourselves, others and human life. All nursing situations involve levels of ethical judgment and decision making, and authenticity permeates every interpersonal encounter. Not everyone is capable of the same degree of authenticity, but it behooves each of us to strive for the highest degree possible.

THE NEED FOR SELF-REFLECTION

It is an existential tenet that the unexamined life is not worth living. Given the types of situations in which we, as nurses, find ourselves on a daily basis, it is clearly necessary that we engage in self-reflection and examine the nature of our nursing encounters. The example of Sartre's anti-Semite is an excellent illustration of how we can become crystallized in a mode of behavior that is totally compliant and unquestioning, with little regard of how this choice impacts on ourselves as well as on the "other" who in this case, is our client. The point is that those of us who strive for authenticity must attempt to be in touch with ourselves as persons and, as much as possible, search for viable alternatives which will be in the client's best interest when ministering nursing care.

Finally, it is important that those of us who strive for authenticity do not shirk professional responsibility; that we do not allow ourselves to be easily swayed toward mediocrity in practice and are concerned as well as involved in those activities that reflect a professional life.

Ethical behavior is a mode of living, a phenomenon that permeates our personal and professional lives. It is our personal lives, however, that affect our professional attitudes and practices. The following quote by Greene, who reminds us that "it must be personal life that is to be changed, not professional attitudes or orientations;" clarifies this point. By substituting the word nurse for teacher, the quote is highly applicable here.

The teacher . . . who pays heed must acknowledge somehow that his effectiveness, like his authenticity, depends to some degree upon the nature of his personal commitment. He must acknowledge that he cannot live in two domains—private and professional. If he has chosen himself to teach, then teaching must become his fundamental project; his means of creating himself.[9]

Thus, in examining the notion of authenticity and its relationship to ethical nursing practice, it becomes clear that ethical behavior is not a unilateral phenomenon. Rather, we engage in ethical practice because we are ethical persons. It is not a question of either/or; it is a matter of what is, or, at least, what we are striving to become.

REFERENCES

1. Levine, M.E. "Nursing Ethics and the Ethical Nurse." *American Journal of Nursing* 77:5 (1977) p. 845.
2. Marcel, G. *The Philosophy of Existentialism* (Secaucus, N.J.: Citadel Press 1956) p. 28. Copyright © 1956. Published by arrangement with Lyle Stuart.
3. Sartre, J.-P. *Portrait of the AntiSemite*. Translated by E. de Mauny (London: Secker and Warbury 1948).
4. Ibid. p. 27.
5. Smith, S. "Outrageous or Outraged: A Nurse Advocate Story." *Nursing Outlook* 28:10 (1980) p. 625. © 1980 American Journal of Nursing Co. Reprinted with permission.
6. Marcel, G. *Being and Having*. Translated by K. Farrer (New York: Harper Torchbooks 1965) p. 47.
7. Marcel, G. *The Mystery of Being: Faith and Reality* vol. 2. Translated by R. Hague (Chicago: Henry Regnery Co. 1951) p. 31.
8. Sartre, J.-P. "Existentialism Is a Humanism" in Kaufmann, W., ed. *Existentialism from Dostoevsky to Sartre* (New York: World Publishing 1956) p. 291.
9. Greene, M. *Existential Encounters for Teachers* (New York: Random House 1967) p. 155. © 1967 Random House, Inc. Reprinted with permission.

Autonomy, Accountability and Nursing Practice

Leah Curtin, M.S., M.A., R.N.
Editor
Nursing Management
Cincinnati, Ohio

THE MOST DRAMATIC way to convey the importance of autonomy is to couch all its ramifications in terms of personal freedom. To deprive individuals of control of their lives is a most brutal rape of the ego. However, recognition and appreciation of the importance of personal freedom do not justify or excuse the individualism gone amuck that often characterizes discussions of autonomy—in or out of the nursing context. Indeed, demands for absolute autonomy—implied or expressed—are a sure impediment to the cooperative team effort necessary for adequate health care delivery. It is incumbent upon all members of the health care professions to reexamine their attitudes and to develop positive and realistic approaches to resolve the tension between concepts of professional and personal autonomy and cooperative, interdependent team action.

THE GENERAL PROBLEM

In debates concerning autonomy, the language of rights frequently is used: rights to self-determination, to personal integrity, to decision making, to equal consideration of interest and so forth. According to Feinberg, "Rights in this category are probably the only ones that are human rights in the strongest sense: unalterable, "absolute," exceptionless and non-conflictable, and necessarily and peculiarly human."[1] Not only has autonomy achieved a sacrosanct place in the philosophical literature, it also has assumed awesome proportions as an essential ingredient of professionalism.

For example, Schechter, writing in the *American Journal of Surgery* claims that a physician has a "right not to have constraints applied to a therapeutic program which he regards as necessary for the patient's welfare or survival."[2] Presumably, this "right" precludes interference from patients, families, nurses, institutions and even statutory bodies.[3] That is, physicians seek *total* control over all matters that affect patients.[4] Largely in response to this attitude among physicians, nurses are demanding professional autonomy and challenging physician and institutional dominance of their practice.

At least part of the problem is the pernicious use of the word autonomy—with all the excess baggage and inappropriate connotations that usually accompany it. The word *autonomy* is derived from two Greek words: *autos* (self) and *nemein* (to hold sway). Thus, the etymological origins of the word infer that it means that "the self holds sway." Modern dictionary definitions of autonomy do not vary significantly from the etymological meaning of the word.[5]

In the philosophy of Kant, autonomy refers to the duty of individuals to govern themselves according to their own reason or, more specifically, to the necessity for human reason to dominate in matters of ethics.[6] Contemporary theories of rights based on Kant's ideal of the autonomy of persons generally hold "that each person is a unique center of reflection and affection and an original source of action."[7] The emphasis is on personal freedom or choice to act or to refrain from acting *within one's own sphere,* "the right to one's *domain,* whether it is one's body, one's life, one's property or one's privacy."[8]

The right to autonomy refers specifically to control of one's own life—not the lives of others. Certainly, any viable contemporary ethic recognizes the social nature of much of human behavior and, at the same time, makes provision for individual freedom. The complexity of modern society and an increasing recognition of human interdependence challenge the legitimacy of any concept of autonomy that is inimical to adequate social cooperation.[9] When autonomy—in or outside of the health care enterprise—is taken to mean that one is answerable only to self and that one is the final arbiter of all action, the results are moral conflict and social chaos. Put quite simply, it is not possible or desirable for the self always "to hold sway" when one lives and works in an interdependent world.

AUTONOMY AND HEALTH CARE

If any one professional or profession is to deliver adequate and humane services to people, all health professions and their practitioners must acknowledge their interdependence—not just with one another, but also with patients or clients, their families and the public at large. Unbridled individualism and insistence on absolute autonomy are antithetical to the achievement of any social goal or even to any civilized intercourse among humans. However, if one denies the central place of the Kantian formulation of moral autonomy, individuals not only would lose control of their own lives but also would be relieved of personal responsibility for decisions made and actions taken.

The task set before us is to find the golden mean between moral autonomy and the cooperative action necessary to contemporary life. One way to go about this task is to distinguish clearly between

---

The task set before us is to find the golden mean between moral autonomy and the cooperative action necessary to contemporary life.

---

those decisions and actions that primarily affect oneself in one's own sphere and those decisions or actions that primarily affect others.

In the first instance, autonomy is legitimate; in the second, a cooperative or social self must replace the autonomous self. (John Stuart Mill taught that individual happiness is bound to the common good. He believed that through education, human beings would learn to identify their personal happiness with the good of society as a whole and thus, progress in human affairs could be made. Ideally then, personal autonomy and cooperative decisions and efforts would not conflict. Actually though, they often do.) However, even

when one accepts the concept of a social self, personal freedom and, hence, responsibility are not sacrificed entirely. Each participant in a group decision is an active part of that decision and each must bear full responsibility for the consequences that flow from it. For example, if one takes part in a group action—perhaps a mob decision to lynch a felon—each person who participated in that action is fully responsible for the felon's death.

One of the greatest dangers of collective decision making (whether this be on a society-wide level or on the more modest level of a hospital committee) is that it will breed a *sense of subservience* to the will of the majority and a *lack of integrity* among individuals.[10] Interdependence requires cooperative decision making, and this in turn requires *voluntary* compliance from each participant in the decision. Voluntary compliance infers that each member of the group assumes the personal duties (1) to participate fully and intelligently in the decision, and (2) to criticize and even oppose decisions when his or her conscience demands it.

VOLUNTARY COMPLIANCE AND THE NURSE

Unfortunately, the situation in the health care system is such that even when nurses are involved in decision making, their compliance is as likely to be *involuntary* as it is to be voluntary. This is the case for a number of reasons: (1) the socialization of nurses to a submissive role;[11] (2) the inconsistent if not chaotic state of nursing education;[12] (3) a lack of appreciation for the knowledge and skills of nurses;[13] (4) the status of nursing as primarily a woman's profession;[14] (5) the oppressive authoritarianism that characterizes hospital bureaucracies;[15] (6) physicians' perceptions of nurses as their obedient assistants;[16] and (7) nurses' perceptions of themselves as powerless, subservient, paramedical personnel.[17] While all the above are well documented and probably accurate, a major part of the problem may be that many nurses are unwilling to assume responsibility for decision making and that nursing has failed to develop an adequate support system for nurses.

Many nursing authors have cited the disparity between what nurses say and what nurses actually do. As Schlotfeldt said in 1965, "The struggle to wrest nursing from the clutches of those who would keep it a field of servitude, rather than a field of professional service, must first be won within the ranks of nursing itself."[18] The lamentable want of cohesiveness and of moral courage among nurses often results in poor patient care. Increasingly, as nurses recognize this fact and as they come to realize their own share of responsibility for it, they are beginning to take action. In addition, as a result of increased education and scholarship,[19] increased appreciation for their own knowledge, skills and contributions and the impact of the feminist movement, nurses have become aware "that they could be independent and decisive, that they could exercise judgment, apply their knowledge, and become involved in policy and decision-making."[20] This emerging assertiveness on the part of nurses coupled with their sincere desire to act as patient advocates[21] is characterized by demands for independent action and an eagerness for autonomy.

However, neither nurses nor patients will be well served by an overzealous (though understandable) insistence on absolute autonomy. What nurses must demand is room for professional decision making about nursing care, and what they must learn to do is to function effectively in an interdependent world. Patients will be no better served if nurses assume dominance than they have been by physicians assuming dominance. *Parity among* the *partners* in the health care endeavor is the key to success.

Physicians' insistence on dominance has placed them under attack from patients' rights organizations,[22] statutory bodies,[23] the courts,[24] other health care professions,[25] and hospital and health care agencies.[26] Quite aside from legal and humanitarian motives, nurses are ill advised to attempt so questionable a course of action. Absolute autonomy (if it ever really existed) is a thing of the past. Care of patients today demands an equitable, compassionate sharing of decision making. This in turn requires a firm grasp of the dynamics and the obligations inherent in group decision making and an understanding of the relationship between moral autonomy and accountability and group action.

AUTONOMY AND GROUP DECISIONS

In general, participation in a group decision obliges one to submit to the authority of the group. It is part of the implied contract one enters into when one consents to participate in the group. There are, of course, exceptions to this obligation. In the context of health care, the patient usually has the right to veto the health care team's decision—primarily because the patient is most directly affected by such decisions and because his or her voluntary compliance usually is essential to the team's success. This may pose certain problems, the exegesis of which is not the subject of this article.

When individuals become members of groups, they assume accountability both to the group and for the group. That is, as a member of a group, a person can be called upon to answer to the group for any actions he or she may take that will affect the group. Moreover, as a member of a group, a person also is answerable for all actions taken by that group (to the individuals most affected by a group decision, to an institution or agency, possibly to statutory bodies or, perhaps, to society at large).

No group member is autonomous: the self cannot "hold sway" because the group's decisions and actions affect more than the self. In addition, participation in a group requires a person voluntarily to assume accountability *to* someone or something other than the self. However, because the individual also has assumed accountability *for* the group, he or she must exercise the responsibilities of freedom within the legitimate structures provided. Therefore, in some instances, it may be necessary for a group member to oppose a group decision. Although noncompliance is not the *right* of any group member, it may be a *duty*.[27] The burden of proof lies with the dissenter.

Anyone who decides to oppose the group's decision must reflect carefully to determine (1) the harm that could result from opposition as weighed against the harm that could result from compliance and (2) the method he or she will use to oppose the decision. Generally, a grave reason is needed to justify noncompliance, and noncompliance always should be preceded by a sincere effort to communicate the facts, reasons and principles that underlie the disagreement. Once this obligation is fulfilled, the dissident has an obligation to use established channels of authority to try to reverse the decision. If this course of action also fails, the dissident *may* be justified in initiating a nonviolent act of moral protest.

However, he or she must be willing to accept whatever disciplinary action that may result from this choice of action. In this manner, the dissident demonstrates respect for both legitimate authority and the integrity of his or her conscience. While it may be necessary to stand alone against the group, such a decision should be weighed carefully and carried out judiciously. Given that the point to be made is important, precipitous or foolish action not only will impede success, it may be used to invalidate the point.

On the other hand, the members of any decision-making body have a duty to weigh carefully any attempt to enforce compliance, particularly on a moral issue. Even if the issue is not a moral one, the decision to use coercion always involves ethical and moral considerations. Within our moral, social and political framework, the high value placed on the principle of liberty sets a presumption against coercion in any form and, most particularly, in matters of conscience.[28]

In fact, a famous American jurist, Harlan Fiske Stone, wrote, "liberty of conscience has a moral and social value which makes it worthy of preservation at the hands of the state. So deep is its significance ... that nothing short of the self-preservation of the state should warrant its violation...."[29] Therefore, if the matter is truly one of conscience, the group rarely should insist upon compliance from a dissident.

To override so strong a prohibition against coercion, certain conditions must be met:[30] (1) an extremely important matter must be at issue; (2) strong evidence is required that the noncompliance of one or even several members of the group will contribute significantly to failure to achieve the group's overridingly important goal; (3) the proportion between the anticipated good and the evil produced by coercion of even one person must be favorable; (4) strong evidence must be produced that the coercion of a group member will provide the desired results; and (5) even if the group decides to impose a decision on group members, the principle of liberty requires that the least coercive means possible be used.

Only after careful consideration of each of these conditions, and after all efforts have been made to secure voluntary compliance, may the group employ any form of coercion. Indeed, it is difficult to imagine too many instances in which the use of coercion is justified.

BACK TO REALITY

Unfortunately, such careful deliberation and exquisite respect frequently are *not* found in group efforts at decision making in the health care system. Only when the conduct of group members demonstrates mutual respect and only when power is equitably distributed can group decision making flourish. Yet if patients are to be served adequately and appropriately in a health care system characterized by rapid change, increasing specialization and sophistication, a multidisciplinary team approach is a practical necessity.

The needs of patients and the demands of the public transcend any one profession's claims to autonomy. Mature team members know that the goal of an interdisciplinary and interdependent team is more important than the "turf" of any one discipline. Although honesty impels one to acknowledge that most nurses are in no position to tackle such a task alone, it also forces one to acknowledge that cries of

---

Cries of inequality, sexism and bureaucratic oppression do not hold water if nurses lack the determination, self–respect and moral courage necessary to establish their roles as full participants in the health care endeavor.

---

inequality, sexism and bureaucratic oppression simply do not hold water if nurses lack the determination, self-respect and moral courage necessary to establish their roles as full participants in the health care endeavor.

Therefore, the disrespect, argumentation, artificial dominance and conflict that typify contemporary interdisciplinary relationships must be overcome. This can be achieved only if antiquated notions of autonomy are replaced with modern ideals of interdependence and cooperation. Interdependence and cooperative action can be achieved only if shared power models replace the monolithic and unilateral power models that typically have controlled the health care system.

If nursing is to establish and maintain itself as an independent profession, a number of steps must be taken. Nurses must continue their efforts to improve nursing education and to establish a consistent entry into practice. Nurses must continue the drive to reform and update nurse practice acts and to lobby extensively for third party reimbursement. Nursing also must upgrade its public image—mature participation in health care decisions on institutional, community, state-wide and national levels is one way to achieve this.

At the same time, nursing must establish recognized support and guidance mechanisms for nurses as they struggle to develop and maintain working relationships with other disciplines. Nurses must learn to walk a thin line firmly identifying their own areas of independent decision making while recognizing and respecting the legitimacy of other disciplines. Despite the difficulties, nurses must maintain attitudes of respect for the education, contributions and services provided by other members of the health care team. Moreover, nurses must have done with fragmentation in their profession and provincialism in their outlook.

The practice of nursing demands that nurses make *professional* judgments—a far cry from inordinate demands for autonomy. Indeed, professional independence consists merely of the freedom to practice one's profession in a responsible and accountable manner. This requires acquisition of the parity and respect necessary for nurses to participate in the group decision making required in contemporary health care. To accomplish these modest goals, nurses must unify now. If they do not nurses never will be free to practice nursing—they will have relinquished control of themselves, nursing practice and the health care system to others—and heated demands for autonomy will not return it to them. Professionalism requires accountability, and professional accountability means that one is answerable to *more* than the self.

REFERENCES

1. Feinberg, J. *Social Philosophy* (Englewood Cliffs, N.J.: Prentice Hall 1973) p. 97.
2. Schechter, P.D. as cited in Macklin, R. "Consent, Coercion and Conflicts of Rights." *Perspectives in Biology and Medicine* (Spring 1977) p. 363.
3. Branson, R. "Distinctions and Priorities among Rights in Health Care" in Smith, D. and Bernstein, L., eds. *No Rush to Judgment* (Bloomington: Indiana University Foundation 1978) p. 203-220.
4. Dachalet, C.Z. "Nursing's Bid for Increased Status." *Nursing Forum* 17:1 (1978) p. 40.
5. *Webster's New Twentieth Century Dictionary* unabridged, 2nd ed. (New York: World Publishing 1966).
6. Kant, I. *Critique of Pure Reason*. Translated by N. Smith. (New York: St. Martin's Press 1965) p. 312.
7. Jonson, A.R. "Right to Health Care Services" in Reich, W.T., ed. *The Encyclopedia of Bioethics* (New York: Free Press 1978) p. 625.
8. Bandman, B. "Option, Rights and Subsistence Rights" in Bandman, E.L. and Bandman, B., eds. *Bioethics and Human Rights* (Boston: Little, Brown 1978) p. 51.
9. Jonson. "Right to Health Care Services."
10. Wellman, C. *Morals and Ethics* (Glenview, Ill.: Scott, Foresman 1975) p. 19.
11. Dachalet. "Nursing's Bid for Increased Status." p. 25.

12. Schlotfeldt, R. "On the Professional Status of Nursing." *Nursing Forum* 8:2 (1974) p. 16-31.
13. National Commission for the Study of Nursing and Nursing Education. *From Abstract into Action* (New York: McGraw-Hill 1973) p. 58.
14. Cleland, V. "Sex Discrimination: Nursing's Most Pervasive Problem." *American Journal of Nursing* 71:8 (1972) p. 1542-1547.
15. Ashley, J.A. *Hospitals, Paternalism and the Role of the Nurse* (New York: Teacher's College Press 1976).
16. Kane, R.L. and Kane, R.A., "Physicians' Attitudes of Omnipotence in a University Hospital." *Journal of Medical Education* 84 (1969) p. 684-690.
17. Dachalet. "Nursing's Bid for Increased Status." p. 23-24.
18. Schlotfeldt, R. "A Mandate for Nurses and Physicians." *American Journal of Nursing* 65 (1965) p. 102-105.
19. Friedson, E. *The Profession of Medicine* (New York: Dodd, Mead and Co. 1973) p. 55.
20. Dachalet. "Nursing's Bid for Increased Status." p. 37-38.
21. Curtin, L. "Human Advocacy: A Philosophical Foundation for Nursing." *Advances in Nursing Science* 1:3 (1979) p. 1-10.
22. Source Inc. *Organizing for Health Care: A Tool for Change* (Washington, D.C.: Beacon Press 1974) p. 1.
23. DHEW Proposed Regulations on Research, 43 Fed. Reg. 1050 (1978).
24. *Natanson v. Kline*, 186 Kan. 393, 350 P.2d(1960); *Schloendorf v. Soc'y of N.Y. Hosps.*, 211, N.Y. 125, 105 N.E. 92, 93 (1914).
25. Perlmutter, D. "Dissent and Conflict in the Health Professions" in Smith and Bernstein, eds. *No Rush to Judgment*. p. 221-237.
26. Source, Inc. *Organizing for Health Care: A Tool for Change.*
27. Whitaker, C. and Coffen, W.S. *Law, Order and Civil Disobedience* (Washington, D.C.: American Enterprise Institute 1967) p. 1.
28. Fried, C. *An Anatomy of Values: Problems of Personal and Social Choice* part III. (Cambridge, Mass.: Harvard University Press 1970) ch. 10-12.
29. Stone, H.F. "The Conscientious Objector." *Columbia University Quarterly* 21 (1919) p. 269.
30. Childress, J.F. "Priorities in the Allocation of Health Resources" in Smith and Bernstein, eds. *No Rush to Judgment*. p. 283-284.

The Concept of Privacy

Marilyn M. Rawnsley, R.N., D.N.Sc.
Associate Dean for Academic
*   Affairs and Professor*
Lienhard School of Nursing
Pace University
Pleasantville, New York

Privacy is a territory that gets to "be our own" in an uneasy truce between ourselves and society.—Arnold Simmel

SCIENCE is amoral. That is, the systematic process of inquiry—including its methods of study and the resultant data—lies outside of the realm of value judgments of right or wrong. There is no tree of knowledge of Good and Evil. What there is, is Actuality—and our attempts to understand it better through scientific investigation. Decisions and actions can be evaluated as moral or immoral but, in itself, information simply exists. It is in the human use of the methods of inquiry and application of the findings that ethical dilemmas arise.

The increasing interest expressed by health professionals about the ethical issues of research and practice reflects both sensitivity to the consciousness-raising messages of the various civil rights movements and recognition of the tremendous impact of an increasingly sophisticated technology. Such concern also testifies to the maturation of the professionals themselves. As they become less awed by the powers of technology they are more able to raise questions about their appropriate use.

A CHAMELEON CONCEPT

Privacy is a salient concern for health professionals, since matters of privacy are inherent in the interactions between them and their clients. For nursing, as a humanistic discipline whose practitioners care for their clients during many intimate and vulnerable moments, participation in the systematic inquiry into the phenomenon of privacy is a relevant responsibility. Moreover, since the hospital environment provides a laboratory of sorts in which invasion of privacy may be epidemic, nursing research that examines the relationships between variables within this context may be not only scientifically enlightening, but even ethically required of us as the discipline responsible for that 24-hour inpatient milieu.

But privacy is a chameleon concept. The Constitution assures Americans of the ideal of privacy as an equal right, and this ideal continues to be reflected in official statements: "The claim to privacy is fragile but persistent; it is as subtle and powerful as the need for personal dignity; it is a fundamental aspect of individual freedom and worth."[1(p8)] Yet our society indicates that privacy is an elitist symbol—for example, the private club, the private beach, the private secretary, the private practice. Is privacy a concept definitive enough to be studied empirically at this time? Beardsley

Our society indicates that privacy is an elitist symbol—for example, the private club, the private beach, the private secretary, the private practice.

addresses its amorphous quality when she notes that statements about privacy tend to be descriptive rather than explanatory: "They do not answer the basic questions of why does privacy exist at all? What functions does it serve? Is it healthy or morbid? Where are its boundaries or zones?"[2(p58)]

THE EVOLUTION OF PRIVACY

Clarification of the dimension of privacy is an essential preliminary to its empirical investigation. Its historical and cultural origins, including the sources of our modern notions of privacy as a legal right, as a social privilege and as a psychological function, need to be considered.

Etymology

The etymology of privacy is a point of departure for understanding the development of this concept. The words *privacy* and *private* are derived from the Latin *privo* which means "to deprive." Its original usage was the military term *private,* which meant literally "to be deprived of status or rank."[3] The stem of *privacy* is *priv,* as is the stem of the word *privilege,* which means a "favoring opportunity."[4] In 1702 Kersey defined *private* as "particular" or "secret," and *privilege* as "a private or particular law."[5]

Anthropology

But 1702 is relatively recent in human history, and there are indications of much earlier origins of this phenomenon. From their cross-cultural anthropological studies, Roberts and Gregor speculated that privacy is a neolithic emergent, since it was negatively correlated with gathering, hunting and fishing societies but more positively associated with herding and agricultural societies, even where there was little political integration.[6]

History

From a historical perspective, Rabkin traces the development of what he calls "inner space" through early and later Greek thought. He notes that the early Bronze Age Greek representations of self depict a series of parts joined together at joints, that the person referred to himself by his own name, and that there seemed to be no concept of the body as a whole. According to Rabkin, the significance of the body concept in later Greek thought is that it provided a container or "space" in which one lived. But this was a physical being who belonged to the state; person and community were fused. As Greek thought evolved, awareness that one was the agent of one's own thoughts and feeling—previously attributed to the gods—also developed. And the psyche, a container within a container, emerged.[7]

From these etymological, anthropological and historical examples, privacy can be postulated to be a psychosocial reality that exists within a matrix of political, technological, psychological and evolutionary phenomena. It is from this concept that the dimensions of privacy in our American culture will be explored.

A LEGAL RIGHT

In the legal realm, privacy as a right has been maturing through a process based on actual court cases. Privacy is thought to be an intangible property emerging from corporeal property and therefore a right to be protected by law.[8] Within the last two decades, the literature from these proceedings has multiplied as the law works its labyrinthian way from particular to precept.

Yet the legal decisions about alleged privacy invasions do little to define its nature. Gross refers to privacy as an "ill-defined embryonic notion" in comparison with "established legal concepts such as trespass, nuisance, defamation and others.... there appears to be no bounds to the areas in which privacy may be found and legal protection sought."[9] Beardsley claims that "the most dependable clue to the content of the norm of privacy in any given society is found in the nature of conduct held to violate privacy."[2] Therefore, from the legal perspective, the boundaries of privacy are defined by their disruption, leaving the essence of the concept to be determined by default.

Consonant with this view is the interpretation of the right of privacy as the right to limit publishing and entertainment media encroachment on the individual, the right to make basic decisions affecting one's own life without government control, and the right to be free of governmental and private surveillance.[10] The issues for current and future health practice and research implied in that statement are considerable!

A SOCIAL PRIVILEGE

Although it should be unnecessary to examine as a privilege that which is by law a right, commonplace observations support the contention that privacy is associated with status and status separation. A relationship between power and privilege has been postulated by Lenski in his second law of distribution, as follows: privilege is largely a function of power, and power determines the distribution of nearly all the surplus (of scarce goods) possessed by a society.[11] If this relationship exists, then one would expect to find privacy unevenly distributed among socio-economic levels, its presence an attribute of affluence, its absence a correlate of control. The following excerpts serve to illustrate the cultural sanction of privacy as a commodity rather than as an equal right:

> Privacy is an object of exchange. It is bought and sold in hospitals, transportation facilities, hotels, theaters, and most conspicuously, in public restrooms....[12]

And,

> Private patients were separated from one another.... The patients in these accommodations did not associate with each other *except on their own terms* ... [In contrast,] patients in multiple bed rooms were acutely aware of suffering and death.[13] [emphasis added]

The final excerpt notes that research itself has violated the privacy of the poor.

> The first large-scale inquiries based on interviewing dealt with slum dwellers, Negroes, immigrants, juveniles on the margin of delinquency, persons with dubious moral standards, et al.—people regarded as not possessing the sensibilities which demand privacy or the moral dignity which requires its respect.[14]

Other authors have cited the affluence of society itself along with its increased industrialization, accelerated technology and sophisticated surveillance techniques as social forces that are undermining privacy.[15,16] But the threats to privacy posed by an affluent society and the notion of privacy as a privilege associated with status and money are not contradictory ideas, since an affluent society does not mean that all the individuals who live in it are affluent. There is a reasonable explanation for this paradox: if affluence and abundance of goods in a society lead to overcrowding in urban areas and increased risks to privacy as described, then privacy may be an increasingly scarce good, a luxury whose accessibility is a function of the power of the individual to purchase it. Within this context, this privacy could be studied as a corollary of Lenski's second law of distribution as previously explained.

A PSYCHOLOGICAL FUNCTION

Privacy as a legal right, privacy as a social privilege; but why be concerned with privacy at all? Is it a human need like sleep or love? The positions on privacy as a psychological need or function can be roughly classified into three groups: (1) those who consider privacy to be an antisocial anachronism, (2) those who think privacy to be a necessary defense mechanism against the pressures of society and (3) those who believe privacy to be a vital condition for personal growth.

Proponents of the first position represent what Weinstein has called a reductionist view. Such views interpret a demand for privacy or removal from the larger group as dysfunctional, a "fall from the perfection of tribal wholeness...[a loss of the] primal experience of fullness."[17(p89-93)] In this view, the consequences of individual privacy on the well-being of the group is of primary concern. Privacy is seen as dysfunctional and as implying a structural inadequacy in the individual.

The second group also assumes a structural inadequacy, but this group ascribes it to the social relations system rather than to the individual. The following excerpt typifies this functionalist point of view:

> Indeed, we retreat to privacy when our expressions of individuality might be too much for our fellow citizens. But that is not the only use we have for privacy. In privacy we can develop, over time, a firmer, better constructed and more integrated position in opposition to dominant social pressures.[18]

Accordingly then, privacy is considered a palliative and a restorative, an opportunity to escape from social stress and to build a stronger defense against its pressures.

In contrast, the third group considers privacy to be germane to the self-actualizing process rather than a retreat due to failure or a withdrawal for repairs. The voluntary, positive aspects of privacy are emphasized: "Privacy, like alienation, loneliness, ostracism and isolation, is a condition of being-apart-from-others. However, alienation is suffered, loneliness is dreaded, ostracism and isolation are borne with resignation or panic, while privacy is sought after."[17(p88)] In the absence of meaningful others or personal purpose only alienation or isolation—but not privacy—can ensue. For privacy requires that there be relevant others from whom one wishes to be apart in order to engage in some fulfilling endeavor. It implies both an appreciation of intimacy and a well-defined self able to enjoy being involved with itself: "Privacy provides the moral context or medium in which arise the higher forms of personal relations, the intimately inviolate and sacred."[19] In summary, privacy is a vehicle in which one travels toward transcendance.

RESEARCH IMPLICATIONS

These three perspectives on the psychological aspects of privacy in addition to the legal, social, and historical dimensions contribute to a broad interpretation of the phenomenon. Still, the concept eludes closure. One reason for this lack of a holistic understanding may be that these dimensions are not additive; privacy includes all of them and yet is something more. "Privacy is the exclusive access of a person to a realm of his own."[20] And where is that realm? What are its generic properties and its delimitations? How can individual privacy zones be assessed? What behaviors indicate deficiencies? What conditions foster the capacity to enjoy and benefit from privacy? Under what conditions is privacy sought? What are the relationships between privacy and creativity, between privacy and perceived locus of control?

Such questions need to be explored in

empirical studies. Typically, research concerned with issues of privacy has focused on related spatial concepts such as territory,[21] interpersonal distance and visual exposure.[22] But research about space and overcrowding that focuses on avoidance patterns appears to be based on an ecological model of space used in studying the effects of overcrowding in animals.[23(p8-11)] The validity of that conceptual model for studying the meaning of human response is questionable.

Perhaps a more relevant framework for investigating the human experience of privacy could be developed from the four functions of privacy postulated by Westin as personal autonomy, emotional release, self-evaluation and limited and protected communication.[23(p32-39)] Moreover, scientific understanding of the nature of privacy might be better advanced through field studies that employ a wide range of descriptive and phenomenological methodologies.

A further caution is warranted. Research into the nature of privacy precipitates an ironic dilemma: when privacy is investi-

Research into the nature of privacy precipitates an ironic dilemma: when privacy is investigated, to some extent it is also invaded.

gated, to some extent it is also invaded. Considerations such as informed consent, protocols for protection of human subjects and avoidance of sampling only those persons who are used to having privacy disrupted might help to minimize unnecessary risks.

But the validity of scientific study depends upon freedom of inquiry. "Behavioral science is obligated to explore all aspects of human behavior to the degree that such inquiry contributes to improved understanding of the nature of man and society."[1(p10)] Improved understanding of the nature of privacy is essential to improved understanding of human nature. And improved understanding of human nature is intrinsic to the theoretical foundations of nursing science.

REFERENCES

1. U.S. Office of Science and Technology. *Privacy and Behavioral Research.* (Washington, D.C.: Government Printing Office, February 1967) p. 8.
2. Beardsley, E.L. "Privacy: Autonomy and Selective Disclosure," in Pennock, J.R., and Chapman, J. eds. *Privacy.* (New York: Atherton Press 1971) p.58.
3. Funk, W. *Word Origins and Their Romantic Stories.* (New York: Grosset & Dunlap 1950) p.230.
4. Kennedy, J. *A Stem Dictionary of the English Language.* (Detroit: Gale Research Co. 1971) p.166.
5. Kersey, J. *A New English Dictionary, 1702.* (Menston, England: The Scolar Press, Ltd. 1969).
6. Roberts, J., and Gregor, T. "Privacy: A Cultural View" in *Privacy.* p. 202.

7. Rabkin, R. *Inner and Outer Space: Introduction to a Theory of Social Psychiatry.* (New York: W.W. Norton & Co. 1970) p. 45-47.
8. Ernst, M., and Schwartz, A. *Privacy: The Right To Be Let Alone.* (New York: Macmillan Co. 1962) p. 47-48.
9. Gross, H. "Privacy and Autonomy" in *Privacy.* p. VII.
10. Pilpel, H. "The Challenge of Privacy" in Reitman, A. ed. *The Price of Liberty.* (New York: W.W. Norton & Co. 1968) p. 23.
11. Lenski, G.E. *Power and Privilege.* (New York: McGraw-Hill 1966) p. 44-45.
12. Schwartz, B. "The Social Psychology of Privacy."

Am J Sociol 73: 61 (May 1968) p. 743.

13. Duff, R., and Hollingshead, A. *Sickness and Society.* (New York: Harper & Row 1968) p. 270-271.

14. Shils, E. "Social Inquiry and the Autonomy of the Individual" in Lerner D., ed. *The Human Meaning of the Social Sciences.* (New York: Meridian Books 1959) p. 116-117.

15. Packard, V. *The Naked Society.* (New York: David McKay 1964) p. 15-43.

16. Van Den Haag, E. "On Privacy" in *Privacy.* p. 163.

17. Weinstein, M. "The Uses of Privacy in the Good Life" in *Privacy.*

18. Simmel, A. "Privacy is Not an Isolated Freedom" in *Privacy.* p. 71-87.

19. Chapman, J. "Personality and Privacy," in *Privacy.* p. 241.

20. Van Den Haag. "On Privacy" in *Privacy.* p. 149.

21. Sommer, R. "Socio-Fugal Space." *Am J Sociol* 72 (May 1967) p. 652-660.

22. Kutner, D.H. "Overcrowding: Human Responses to Density and Visual Exposure." *Human Relations* 26 (1973) p. 31-50.

23. Westin, A.F. *Privacy and Freedom.* (New York: Atheneum Press, 1967).

Ethical Issues and Procedural Dilemmas in Measuring Patient Competence

Virginia Kilpack, RN, MSN
Clinical Nurse Specialist in Neurology and
* Neurosurgery*
Department of Nursing
Dartmouth Hitchcock Medical Center
Hanover, New Hampshire

IS THERE a line between competence and incompetence, or is the difference an arbitrary determination? Frequently, the determination of incompetence may appear arbitrary because the rationale for this decision making is not clear or not revealed. The definition of incompetence often varies from caregiver to caregiver within the same setting. Because nursing is concerned with ensuring the right of the patient to make decisions, uncertainty arises when there are questions about the patient's ability to make decisions or when the patient makes decisions that will not promote health and that predictably have serious sequelae. Some of the confusion in knowing how to intervene in these circumstances may relate to the fact that the concept of competence is multidimension-

The author wishes to thank Anne-Marie Barron, MSN, RN, formerly Psychiatric Liaison Clinical Nurse Specialist, Dartmouth-Hitchcock Medical Center and Bernard Gert, PhD, Stone Professor of Intellectual and Moral Philosophy, Dartmouth College, who has an NEH-NSF Sustained Development Award ISP-8018088 A01, for their assistance in the preparation of this article.

al; it is a social and legal concept as well as a medical and psychiatric concept. Divergent views can be seen in the models of competency measurement as found in the literature of law, medicine, and philosophy.

ALTERNATIVE CONCEPTIONS OF COMPETENCY

Models from psychiatry

Roth et al[1] reviewed competency tests as found in psychiatric literature and judicial commentary and organized them into five separate categories. Some of the categories showed overlap and some were inferred from the literature.

Test 1—Evidencing a choice. This test for competency requires the patient to show preference for or against treatment. The patient could be considered competent even if help is sought to make the treatment decision. When the patient is verbally silent, behavior is evaluated to judge the direction of the response; ie, if there is compliance with the treatment requirements when every opportunity is given for refusal of each modality offered, the patient is considered to be evidencing a choice and, therefore, to be competent. This test may not reveal the patient's understanding of the choice made; therefore, it is a low-level test in regard to determining if a patient makes an informed decision. Examples of patients who would be judged incompetent by this test are those who are unconscious, delirious, or psychiatrically mute.

Test 2—Reasonable outcome of choice. This test focuses on the outcome of the decision-making process, rather than the ability to make a decision. The test requires the patient to make the right or "reasonable" decision to be considered competent. The reasonable decision is the one that a reasonable person in like circumstances would make. Judicial decisions usually favor preservation of health, and that bias is commonly held by health care providers; thus, the patient whose outcome of choice is congruent with this bias is always considered competent. It is easy to see how this test could be used to determine that the patient is incompetent when there is refusal to acquiesce to treatment. With this test, the outcome of choice, not the patient, is evaluated. The circular nature of the test reduces its value for clinical use. It makes no contribution to an understanding of the decision-making process of the patient, and it has the potential to erode personal autonomy.

Test 3—Choice based on rational reasons. In this test the reasons for the patient's decision are evaluated to determine if they are "rational." Examples from the literature reviewed by Roth et al equated rational with the absence of mental illness, and Roth et al implied that mental illness is interpreted as disordered cognitive function, ie, delusion and/or delirium. Like the first test, this is a very low-level test of competence. Even for patients with mental illness, it is usually not possible to prove that the mental illness was responsible for the patient's treatment decision; for example, a delusional patient may reject extensive surgery out of fear, which is a normal reaction and not the result of the delusional state. This test offers little conceptual clarity about how to evaluate the quality of the patient's thinking. A decision in favor of treatment usually does not stimulate a concern for competence.

Test 4—Ability to understand. This test is most consistent with the current legal and ethical principles of informed consent and requires the patient to answer questions or show some understanding of risks, benefits, and alternatives to treatment. Understanding does not have to be perfect for the patient to be considered competent. The level of understanding required to pass this test cannot be precisely determined because few attempts at quantifying understanding have been made.[2] Meisel and Roth[3] reviewed numerous studies of informed consent to ascertain how the concept of understanding was made operational. Few hard data were found; the primary weakness of these studies was the limited reporting of the information given to patients when informed consent was obtained. Unfortunately, recall seemed to be equated with understanding by many investigators.

This test, like test 3, emphasizes only the cognitive ability of the patient to compre-

Table 1. Measurement of patient competency to consent to or refuse treatment

Test/criteria for competence	Criteria for incompetence
Roth et al[1]	
Test 1—Evidencing a choice	No treatment choice is manifested
Test 2—Reasonable outcome of choice	Treatment choice is not like that of reasonable person
Test 3—Choice based on rational reasons	Cognitive disorder is present
Test 4—Ability to understand	Cognitive facts are not understood
Test 5—Actual understanding	Treatment situation is not completely understood or integrated
Meisel[2]	

Status tests
  Permanent conditions
  Temporary conditions
  Transitory/subjective characteristics
	There is deviation from hypothetical average person

Functional tests Absence of decision	No treatment choice is manifested
Nature of decision-making process	Unacceptable means of making decision are used
Nature of decision	Treatment choice is not in accordance with verifiable standard
Lack of understanding of informed consent	Information relevant to informed consent is not understood
Beauchamp and Childress[3]	
Understanding the treatment	Rational reasons are not used to meet criteria
Weighing risks and benefits of treatment	
Making decision in light of such knowledge	

Table 1 *(continued)*

Test/criteria for competence	Criteria for incompetence
Culver et al[4]	
Patient knows—	Criteria are not met
Physician believes patient is ill and needs treatment	
Physician believes certain treatment will help illness	
Patient is being asked to decide about treatment	
Culver and Gert[5]	
Completely incompetent	Patient is an infant, severely retarded or senile, comatose, or can identify only immediate needs
Competent to give or refuse simple consent	Patient can comprehend only part of treatment situation
Competent to give or refuse valid consent	

[1]Roth L, Meisel A, Lidz C: Tests of competency to consent to treatment. *Am J Psychiatry* 1977;134:279–284.
[2]Meisel A: Legal overview, in Reatig N (ed): *Competency and Informed Consent,* US Department of Health and Human Services publication No. (NIMH) 81-23. National Institute of Mental Health, 1981, pp 32–71.
[3]Beauchamp T, Childress J: *Principles of Biomedical Ethics.* New York, Oxford Univ Press, 1979, pp 62–85.
[4]Culver C, Ferrell R, Green R: *ECT and Special Problems of Informed Consent. Am J Psychiatry* 1980;135:586–591.
[5]Culver C, Gert B: *Philosophy in Medicine.* New York, Oxford Univ Press, 1982, pp 42–63.

hend the treatment facts (or information of equivalent intricacy). No significance is attributed to the way in which the patient weighs the facts presented. Examples of patients who might be considered incompetent by this test are those with mental retardation of such a degree that they are unable to comprehend the situation, those with delirium, and those with levels of drug intoxication that would interfere with comprehension.

Test 5—Actual understanding. This test is similar to test 4, but it adds the obligation that the health care provider instruct the patient and then ascertain if the patient really understood the full meaning of the treatment information. Criteria for performance of this test are not defined; the health care provider is expected to make a genuine effort to educate the patient about the total treatment situation and its complexities. In general, the amount of understanding needed by the patient is potentially greater than that required in test 4. This high-level test of competence is important in situations when patients agree to treatment that carries high risk or when they refuse beneficial treatment with negligible risk.

Consider an alert, elderly cancer patient who requests the alleviation of suffering and support in maintaining respectability during the last days or months of life but who will not accept nursing interventions to meet these desires because of the presence and threat of pain. With the actual understanding test, it is uncertain if the patient meets the requirements for competence. The patient appears to be sensitive to the realities of a fast-approaching death but will not accept measures to facilitate clearly stated goals. The omission of these nursing measures could cause significant harm to the patient. Test 5 highlights the conceptual difficulties in measuring the understanding of the patient and the personal meaning of that understanding. There is obvious potential for disagreement in patient evaluation. However, this test is intended to be comprehensive; it is meant to measure more than the patient's knowledge of the facts presented.

In summary, Roth and associates believe that the competency test used will often be some combination of these five tests, because no single test will encompass all biases held by the evaluator (Table 1).

Model from law

Meisel[4] provides a legal model regarding what it means to be competent to make treatment decisions as required by the doctrine of informed consent (Table 1). However, the focus of this model is incompetence and it is defined in terms of *status and functional tests.* A patient who has a certain status or lacks a certain functional ability would not be qualified to participate in the treatment decision-making process. Persons who deviate from the "average" and have one of the following characteristics would be considered incompetent: a permanent condition, ie, severe mental retardation; a temporary condition such as intoxication; or a transitory or subjective characteristic such as peculiar behavior or appearance. These status tests provide a quick but limited measurement of the patient.

The functional tests of incompetency specify the deficits in the decision-making process that prohibit the patient from making autonomous decisions. In the test for *absence of a decision,* the patient can be deemed incompetent when there is failure to make a choice about treatment, as in the test of Roth et al for evidencing a choice.

In the test for the *nature of the decision-making process* a patient is judged incompetent in the following circumstances.

- There is failure to give reasons supporting a treatment choice.
- No rational reasons are given to support a treatment choice. (Rational reason is defined as the use of reality-based information but may include nonobjective facts reflecting a patient's preference. This definition is different from that in the test of Roth et al of choice based on rational reasons.)
- There is no evaluation of risks versus benefits; this is similar to the test of Roth et al for *ability to understand.*

The test for the *nature of a decision* is used to evaluate the outcome of the decision-making process and determines the patient to be incompetent when the choice does not match certain standards, such as the physician's recommendation or the hypothetical standard of the reasonable person, like the test of Roth et al for *reasonable outcome of choice.*

Like the test of Roth et al for ability to understand, the test for *lack of understanding of informed consent* measures incompetence by (1) actual understanding (observation that the patient lacks cognitive ability to understand the information disclosed) or by (2) ability to understand (inferential determination, perhaps from such sources as informal conversation or an intelligence score). These functional tests do not presume that a mentally ill patient is incompetent; rather, the test used determines the cognitive abilities to be assessed. The choice of a test usually reflects the tester's perception of what needs to be understood; thus, the tester's values significantly influence the determination of patient incompetence.

Meisel recommends starting with the test for the understanding component, when informed consent for research participation is sought. This test lacks the extremes of values intrinsic in the tests for the absence and the nature of a decision; is consistent with the implied meaning of consent; and meets federal regulations.[5] These functional tests have many of the same strengths and weaknesses as similar tests described by Roth et al, but Meisel's emphasis is to define incompetence as a means of knowing or presuming that persons outside this definition are competent to give informed consent.

Model from philosophy

Beauchamp and Childress,[6] who have philosophical interests in ethics, describe the concept of competence as it relates to

---

The choice of a test of patient competence usually reflects the tester's perception of what needs to be understood; thus, the tester's values significantly influence the determination of incompetence.

---

informed consent in a biomedical context. They believe competence to consent is a precondition of acting voluntarily. Conditions external and internal to a patient may limit voluntary action, but it is usually the internal conditions that raise concern about competence. The investigators introduce the concepts of limited and intermittent competence, highlighting the fact that a person's ability to make decisions can vary over time and that an individual can be competent to make certain decisions but incompetent to make others. For example, a person with a delirium, a condition in which mental status characteristically fluctuates, might be intermittently competent, that is, competent during the periods of time when mental status was not impaired. A person who has generally exhibited normal behavior except in relation to circumscribed delusional thinking might have limited competence.

These authors cite an example of a man who behaves normally in most areas of living but engages in self-mutilating behavior because he believes God is asking him to sacrifice himself for the good of humankind. To determine that this individual or the delirious person is totally incompetent to make any treatment decisions limits the self-determination of both in unnecessary and unjustifiable ways; yet, both examples demonstrate a lack, at times, of the ability to understand sufficiently to give informed consent.

In recent years, there has been a major question in relation to determination of criteria for assessing competence. Beauchamp and Childress state that conventional criteria isolate various abilities to understand information and to reason about the consequences of personal

actions. Legal definitions of competency
vary, but these authors point out that one
or more of the following three criteria are
generally considered to be essential by the
courts[6(p69)]:
- "capacity to reach a decision based on
rational reasons" (similar to test 3 of
Roth et al);
- "reaching a reasonable result through a
decision" (similar to test 2 of Roth et
al); and
- "the capacity to reach a decision at all"
(possibly related to test 1 of Roth et
al).
Combining these criteria, Beauchamp
and Childress state that a person is competent only if decisions are made on the basis
of rational reasons and that in biomedical
contexts this criterion subsumes that the
person must be able to (1) understand the
treatment, (2) weigh its risks and benefits,
and (3) make a decision in light of such
knowledge, even if the choice is not to use
the information given. These authors do
not identify the behaviors that demonstrate
the evaluation of information in decision
making, and they only imply that all three
of their criteria must be met to judge an
individual competent (Table 1).

Model from psychiatry and religion

Culver et al[7] are from the disciplines of
psychiatry and religion, and they explain
competence by the use of narrow behavioral referents. They say patients are competent to decide about treatment when the
following minimal criteria are met: (1) the
patient knows the physician believes he or
she is ill and needs treatment, (2) the
patient knows the physician believes that a
certain treatment will relieve the illness,
and (3) the patient knows he or she is being
asked to decide about this treatment.[7] The
patient's realization is primarily based on
awareness of the current situation and the
patient's ability to give and receive communication.

The authors point out that in clinical
practice, the patient who refuses treatment
believed to be necessary and/or beneficial
by the health care professional often is
deemed incompetent solely because treatment is refused. The labeling of incompetence allows the health care professional to
think that it is in the best interest of the
patient for the professional to insist on
certain treatment for an individual who is
unable to make decisions autonomously.
Culver et al make a salient point: judgment
about patient competence should be made
independently of the patient's treatment
decision. Because the determination of
competence indicates how a discussion of
treatment will proceed, it is essential that
the health care provider recognize personal
bias toward treatment and separate the
evaluation of competence from a treatment decision.

These investigators recommend that
once a patient has made a decision, the
quality of the decision itself must be
assessed to determine if it is rational or
irrational. Except in unusual cases it would
be considered irrational for the patient to
act in a manner that is contrary to personal
desires, in regard to such factors as freedom, pleasure, and suffering.[8]

Imagine that a post operative patient
who has had no previous drug-related
problems refuses to be medicated for pain
following surgery. The patient rejects medication because of fear of drug addiction
despite efforts at education about narcot-

ics. Although the criteria of the authors indicate that there may be no reason to question the patient's competence to make decisions regarding care, it is possible that the decision to reject pain relief results from an inappropriately strong fear, assuming there is no factual disagreement with the physician. According to Culver et al, the patient would be viewed as competent to make this decision, but the quality of the decision rendered would be considered irrational. Even when the quality of a decision is considered irrational, these authors say the decision should be respected, unless there are compelling reasons to override it, such as life-threatening or highly deleterious sequelae.

Professional behavior in relation to a patient's right to make a decision is generally clear when (1) the patient has been determined to be incompetent by most of the tests discussed here or (2) the patient is competent and making rational decisions. Competently made irrational decisions, though infrequently encountered by the health care professional, can present difficult problems. Culver et al offer clarification in this situation by making a distinction between incompetence and irrationality, allowing competent patients to make irrational decisions. It may be necessary and justifiable[9,10] to overrule some refusals of treatment, but it would not always be based on the grounds that the patient was incompetent (Table 1).

Model from psychiatry and philosophy

Culver and Gert[11] write primarily for people in medicine who have philosophical interests. They distinguish between two levels of incompetence in relation to valid consent (Table 1). The first category of patients would include those who are unable to give or refuse even simple consent (eg, infants, patients in coma, or severely retarded patients). The authors indicate further that it would be universally acknowledged as justifiable and even required morally for someone else to be appointed to make decisions for them.

Also included in this category are patients who are less than totally incompetent, who may be significantly limited in cognitive abilities but able to identify immediate needs and concerns such as hunger or discomfort. They would, however, not understand questions or concerns unrelated to immediate stimuli and therefore they would not understand that they are being asked for consent. Culver and Gert refer to patients in this category as being *incompetent to give simple consent*. This group of patients also would need others appointed to make their decisions for them.

The second category of patients these authors describe are those who are *incompetent to give valid consent*. These patients could understand that they were being asked to consent to a treatment and could actually give consent or refusal, but they would be unable to understand or appreciate the information necessary to give valid consent. Examples of patients in this category would be mildly delirious, mildly retarded, or mildly demented patients who may have only partial grasp of the situation or those who have delusions directly related to giving or withholding consent, eg, patients with paranoid belief that the health care providers are plotting to harm them. Culver and Gert describe these patients as being incompetent to give valid consent but competent to give simple consent.

There is an important difference between the two levels of incompetence. For those patients incompetent to give simple consent, another person should be appointed to make decisions for them. The health care provider would not be in the position of overruling this patient's decision because nothing the patient does is viewed as giving or refusing consent. For those patients considered incompetent to give valid consent but competent to give or refuse simple consent, the situation is more intricate. Neither a consent nor a refusal of consent could be considered valid, since the patient lacks the ability to

---

Culver and Gert believe it is a very serious matter to give treatment without the consent of the patient, even when the patient is not considered competent to give valid consent.

---

understand and appreciate the information being considered, so, again, a guardian should be appointed to decide on behalf of the patient.

A problem arises if the patient has given a simple refusal and the guardian disagrees with that refusal. These authors believe it is a very serious matter to give treatment without the consent of the patient, even when the patient is not considered competent to give valid consent. They advocate taking simple refusals of consent to treatment very seriously and overruling them only in special situations, when not treating

the patient would involve significant harm. On the other hand, if the patient gives a simple consent to treatment and the guardian disagrees with that consent, Culver and Gert presume that the guardian is simply protecting the patient's interests.

To be competent to give *valid consent* the patient must be presented with sufficient information to make an informed decision and must be able to understand and appreciate that information. The aspect of understanding and appreciating the information is crucial. If anxiety results in inability to integrate all of the treatment information, the patient would not have adequate information and could not give valid consent. Because assessing the understanding requires being with and talking with the patient at some length, Culver and Gert suggest that, in an inpatient setting, the nurse is often in the best position to determine whether the patient has adequate information on which to base the decisions for treatment.

ANALYSIS OF MODELS

Major likenesses and differences are apparent in the preceding models. Tests 1, 3, and 4 of Roth et al are similar to the criteria used by Beauchamp and Childress to determine competence. In addition, Beauchamp and Childress recommend that judgments about competence take place within a specific context, so that an individual is not considered to be totally competent or totally incompetent. They encourage the establishment of criteria for determining competence, while recognizing that the initial choice of criteria establishes that certain abilities are essential.

The criteria of Culver et al show a

likeness only to test 1 of Roth et al. Culver et al do not specify the process that should be used to arrive at a treatment decision, because they assess competence prior to and independently of the patient's treatment choice. In addition, they define a difference between incompetence and irrationality. This adds precision to an understanding of the quality of the treatment decision because it allows the competent patient to remain competent, even when an irrational decision is made. This is a significant perspective because the patient judged incompetent would still be incompetent, even if there was subsequent consent to treatment.

Only Roth et al allow for test 2; this test evaluates the decision made by the patient but never evaluates the patient and would be regarded as a test of rationality, not competence, by Culver et al. Test 2 encourages the health care provider to enforce personal values instead of those of the patient; it assumes that the result is all-important. Content comparable to test 2 of Roth et al was found only in Meisel's test, nature of decision; however, Meisel comes from the discipline of law, in which it is common to measure action against a normative standard. Both tests appear to be inappropriate for use in the evaluation of patient competence.

Test 5 is thought to have the greatest reliability of the five tests of Roth et al, even though what constitutes the depth of actual understanding is not completely clear. Deficits in understanding could be ascribed to the health care provider as well as the patient. The explanation by Culver and Gert of competence for valid consent has a similarity to test 5; they specifically point out that valid consent means full

attention must be directed to the patient to ensure that consent is truly informed consent, because it has been personalized. Culver and Gert expand the discussion of competence by specifying two levels of incompetence, a distinction not mentioned by the other authors. This distinction guides the health care provider in knowing that it is appropriate for some incompetent patients to make a treatment choice, even though the choice would not be truly an informed one, and in knowing what considerations should follow.

The lowest level tests of competency are test 1 of Roth et al; the minimal criteria used by Culver et al; and those tests used by Culver and Gert to determine competence to give or refuse simple consent. The highest level tests of competency are test 5 of Roth et al; the tests used by Culver and Gert to determine ability to give valid consent; and the three criteria of Beauchamp and Childress.

The bias of health care providers is slanted toward treatment; therefore, it is imperative that the competency test applied is not selected on this basis. In classifying competence to consent to or refuse treatment, Culver and Gert guarded against this bias by using specific competency descriptions to place the patient in one of three categories that determine whether the giving or refusing of consent will be valid. It is the classification of competence that makes the work of Culver and Gert more helpful than that of Culver et al; criteria of Culver et al for competence results in some ambiguities when competence is limited or fluctuating, and it is not clear how this should be evaluated when valid consent is determined.

The literature reviewed shows how difficult it is to have congruence on what it means to be competent, because of the variableness and doubtfulness of how incompetence is to be determined. Most efforts at defining competence have been directed toward consent to treatment rather than consent to research.[4,12-14]

NURSING AND COMPETENCY ASSESSMENT

Although nurses support and guide patients daily in fulfilling diagnostic treatment requirements, this is not done with ease when patients begin refusing to comply with protocols of health care. The nursing literature reveals no model to follow when there is a need to assess patient competence in order to know whether a paternalistic posture would be justified[15] or whether the patient's sovereign state should be respected. From a legal view, persons are considered competent until it is determined otherwise by a judicial hearing; however, clinical situations that require a nurse to make a competency assessment are a reality and are often of a pressing nature.

Illness does not necessarily distort the wishes of the true self; therefore, a person cannot be judged incompetent only because personal choices change after the start of a sickness. The autonomy of individuals is seriously respected by nurses, but a paradigm is needed for offering this protection when a patient's competency is being challenged.

Studies in nursing have not described the communication of nurses to patients about (independent) nursing treatments or the effects when these interventions are refused. This issue is complex because the nurse assists the patient with nursing prescriptions and the medical regimen, and the patient can refuse either or both of these, thereby risking detrimental consequences. This could result in the need to manage competing values of treatment, and it is uncertain if there is nursing consensus on the competency model to apply.

As the disease process may affect the patient's mental capacity, so also can interpersonal factors or the real or imagined features of a health care facility.[16] A high level of awareness is needed by the nurse to distinguish a competency assessment issue from these other effects. The preceding models of competency determination provide some conceptual understanding of how to act in a knowledgeable way, lifting moral choice out of an intuitive base. Judgments of patient competence can be based on understood concepts and are not to be confused with bias held by the health care provider. Although many patients are competent to make decisions about their nursing care and health care, it is important to address those borderline areas of competency that provoke uncertainty and need formulation by nursing.

REFERENCES

1. Roth L, Meisel A, Lidz C: Tests of competency to consent to treatment. *Am J Psychiatry* 1977;134:279-284.

2. Olin G, Olin H: Informed consent in voluntary mental hospital admissions. *Am J Psychiatry* 1975;132:934-941.

3. Meisel A, Roth L: What we do and do not know about informed consent. *JAM* 1981;246:2473-2477.

4. Meisel A: Legal overview, in Reatig N (ed): *Competency and Informed Consent,* US Department of Health and Human Services publication No. (NIMH) 81-23. National Institute of Mental Health, 1981, pp 32-71.

5. US Department of Health and Human Services: Final Regulations Amending Basic HHS Policy for the Protection of Human Research Subjects. *Federal Register* 1981;46 (Jan):8366-8392.

6. Beauchamp T, Childress J: *Principles of Biomedical Ethics.* New York, Oxford Univ Press, 1979, pp 62-85.

7. Culver C, Ferrell R, Green R: ECT and Special Problems of Informed Consent. *Am J Psychiatry* 1980;135:586-591.

8. Gert B: *The Moral Rules,* paperback ed 2. New York, Harper Torchbooks, 1975.

9. Gert B, Culver C: The Justification of Paternalism. *Ethics* 1979;89:199-210.

10. Childress J: *Who Should Decide?* New York, Oxford Univ Press, 1982.

11. Culver C, Gert B: *Philosophy in Medicine.* New York, Oxford Univ Press, 1982, pp 42-63.

12. Applebaum PS, Roth L: Competency to consent to research. *Arch Gen Psychiatry* 1982;39:951-958.

13. Roth L, Lidz C, Meisel A, et al: Competency to decide about treatment or research. *Int J Law Psychiatry* 1982;5:29-50.

14. Annas GJ, Glantz LH, Katz BF: *Informed Consent to Human Experimentation: The Subject's Dilemma.* Cambridge, Mass, Ballinger Publishing Co, 1977, pp 33-38.

15. Marchewka A: When is Paternalism Justifiable? *Am J Nurs* 1983;83:1072-1073.

16. Applebaum PS, Roth L: Clinical issues in the assessment of competency. *Am J Psychiatry* 1981;138:1462-1467.

Rethinking the Nurse's Role in "Do Not Resuscitate" Orders: A Clinical Policy Proposal in Nursing Ethics

Roland R. Yarling
PhD Candidate
Department of Ethics and Society
University of Chicago
Chicago, Illinois

Beverly J. McElmurry, RN, EdD, FAAN
Professor
University of Illinois
College of Nursing
Chicago, Illinois

THE QUESTION OF when to use and when not to use cardiopulmonary resuscitation (CPR) is a problem familiar to the practitioners of nursing and medicine. It characterizes the complex issues that have developed in health care as a result of the advance of medical technology and the emergence of patient autonomy. It is now technically possible to do many things that from a moral perspective sometimes should not be done.

In the last few years, it has been common for hospitals to establish institutional policy in regard to "do not resuscitate" (DNR) orders, although many still do not have such a policy. These policies address specific questions including

- the conditions under which a DNR decision may be made (the terminal status of the patient),
- who should make the decision when the patient is competent (the patient),
- who should make it when the patient is not competent (usually the health care team and the family),

- who should implement it (the physician), and
- how it should be implemented (in writing).

Frequently, it is the nursing staff in a hospital who requests that such policy be established because DNR orders have long been a source of conflict and frustration for nurses. The problem has been discussed repeatedly in the nursing literature from a nursing perspective.[1-8] These discussions usually focus on the problem of physicians who give only verbal orders, order "slow codes," will not honor a patient's desire not to be resuscitated, write an order for a competent patient without consulting the patient, and/or do not communicate with the nursing staff about the orders they write. It is in response to such problems that nurses have urged the adoption of a responsible institutional policy to regularize decisions and procedures pertaining to DNR orders.

Given the relatively widespread policy activity by hospitals on this matter in the late 1970s, it might have been concluded that the corner had been turned and that the problem was being resolved. Whatever illusions may have been entertained in that regard were effectively dispelled with Curtin's 1979 editorial.[9] More letters were received in response to that editorial than to any editorial in the history of the journal, according to the editor. Curtin said that CPR is often misused and that conflict over the matter frequently puts the nurse in a difficult position. The issue is still being hotly contested in hospitals. It takes only a 1-page editorial to unleash the frustration of nurses. Many hospitals, regardless of size, still have no DNR policy, and even in those that have a policy, problems continue largely because physicians frequently

disregard it even when it has been approved by the medical board.

Furthermore, the issue has symbolic importance. The conflict between nursing and medicine around this issue is paradigmatic of the general nature of the relationship of nursing and medicine historically. Medical authoritarianism and unjustifiable institutional constraints have long served to impede the practice of nursing as defined by the profession and to render nurses less able to act responsibly vis-à-vis the needs and rights of their patients. The conflict around DNR orders is a microcosm of the larger picture.

WHY ONLY THE PHYSICIAN

This suggests that a more fundamental reassessment of the situation is in order. What kind of a decision is a DNR decision? It is *not* a medical decision, although it usually follows from a medical judgment concerning the irreversible nature of the patient's disease. The DNR decision must be clearly distinguished from a medical judgment about the irreversibility of a disease. This medical judgment is a necessary, but not a sufficient, condition for the DNR decision. It is *not* a *nursing* decision, even though the nurse as well as the physician may need to assist the competent patient in reaching an authentic decision about what he or she chooses to have done. It is *not* a *legal* decision, but it has strong legal entailments. It is a *moral* decision; therefore, it properly belongs to the patient.

In the case of an incompetent patient, it is still a moral decision and should usually be made by the family in consultation with the health care team. If there is no family, the decision rests by default with the health care team, including the physician, nurse, and clergy. The important point to be made here, however, is that the majority of patients could make this decision for themselves if those working with the patient would initiate a discussion of the question before the patient deteriorates into incompetence. Because such discussions can be difficult, they are too often postponed until the patient becomes incompetent, and then the difficulties of making the decision for the patient must be faced.

To assert that DNR decisions are moral decisions rather than medical, nursing, or legal decisions does not mean that medical, nursing, and legal decisions do not have a moral dimension. The point is that a DNR decision should not be based on extraneous criteria but rather on the moral values of the patient—values concerning the meaning, sanctity, and quality of life.

The decision is a moral decision because the criteria for the decision are moral values. The nature of a decision is not determined by its consequences but by its criteria. For instance, a DNR decision entails the withholding of medical treatment, and it will have consequences for the medical status of the patient, but that does not make it a medical decision. So also, a decision of Congress not to provide funding for a totally implantable artificial heart for everyone who might reasonably be judged to benefit significantly from it would have tremendous implications for the field of cardiology and for the medical status of cardiac patients. However, such a decision would not be a medical decision. It would be a political-moral decision based on political and moral criteria.

Thus, a DNR decision, which is rightly based on moral considerations such as the

value of life itself, the quality of life under given conditions, and the acceptance or denial of the imminence of death by the patient, is a moral decision, not a medical decision. Such moral decisions involve questions of values that are not related to the special expertise of the physician, the nurse, or the attorney. The proper basis for their resolution is the patient's value system. Therefore, it is a decision that belongs to the patient.[10]

If a DNR decision is not a medical decision, a nursing decision, or a legal decision, but a moral decision to be made by the patient, what is the logic of the situation that dictates that the decision of the patient be implemented by a physician? Why should the physician alone be the person designated in DNR policies to write the DNR order?

The question pertains to whether the patient is competent or incompetent. Although the patient is referred to as the decision maker in DNR situations, the arguments that follow apply equally to situations in which the patient is incompetent and the DNR decision must be made by the family and/or the health care team.

The most obvious recourse in response to the question is the legal requirements. It may be argued that writing orders, DNR orders in this case, is, by law, a physician function. The law on this question varies from state to state, but the Illinois Nursing Act does not say that writing orders is not a nursing function. It says that nursing shall not "include those acts of medical diagnosis or prescription of therapeutic or corrective measures which are properly performed only by physicians ...," (*The Illinois Nursing Act of 1975*, Ill Rev Stat tit 91, §35.32–35.57), but it does not designate which acts of medical diagnosis or prescription are properly performed only by physicians. There is clearly much room for discussion in Illinois.

Furthermore, regardless of the wording of specific nursing acts in various states, legal requirements are often nothing more than a recognition of the way things have usually been done. This is what has been referred to as making medical law on the basis of the "may I do you?" syndrome. The physician goes to the court and says, "May I do thus and so?" The court says, "Do you, ie, the medical community, ordinarily do thus and so?" The physician says, "We do." The court says, "Then you may." According to this model, the law deals more with the issue of what is than what ought to be. Appeal is implicitly made to the principle of the existing community standard of care.

Mill and Mill cogently observed that "laws and systems of polity always begin by recognizing the relation they find already existing between individuals. They convert what was a mere physical fact into a legal right, and give it the sanction of society."[11(p130)] But in so doing, the law may well sanction unjust situations.

From a moral point of view, can any good reasons be given for the status quo? Can a law or policy that designates the physician as the only person who can write a DNR order be morally justified? It is commonly stated and widely held that the physician in charge of a patient is fully responsible for the patient's full treatment and care. But this is not the case either in fact or law.

The physician in charge is responsible only for the patient's *medical* diagnosis and treatment, much of which must be implemented by the nurse; the nurse, on the other hand, is responsible for the patient's *nursing* diagnosis and treatment (*Darling v Charleston Community Memorial Hospital*, 50 [Ill App 2d 253; 200 NE 2nd 149; (1965) *aff'd;* 33 Ill 2d 327; 211 NE 2d 253 [1964] *cert denied;* and *Utter v United Hospital Center, Inc, and Lawrence Mills*, 236 SE [2d] 213 [WVa] [1977]),[12] in addition to implementing the physician's orders (or more properly, the physician's prescriptions). And nursing diagnosis and treatment are based on independent nursing judgments. If responsibility for the patient's diagnosis, treatment, and care falls primarily into two domains—the physician's responsibility for *medical* diagnosis and treatment and the nurse's responsibility for *nursing* diagnosis and treatment—the logical question is, again, why should this decision of the patient be implemented by the physician?

One viewpoint is that this task rightly belongs to the physician because the patient's decision is based on the medical judgment of the physician about the irreversibility of the disease. To the contrary, however, this medical judgment is not the *basis* of the patient's decision but is a *precondition* of the decision, like the disease itself. The proper *basis* of the patient's decision is the value system of the patient.

Another viewpoint is that the physician should write the order because the physician is usually the person to discuss the question with the patient. However, this assumption is questionable both in terms of what does happen and in terms of what should happen. In fact, patients probably discuss this matter more often with the nursing staff than with the medical staff.

With reference to what should happen, the best person to discuss the matter with the patient may or may not be the responsible physician because the decision is a moral decision based on the patient's value system. Technical skill does not translate into moral wisdom, so the best person to talk with the patient may be the physician, the nurse, clergy, a family member, or any other person with the appropriate sensitivity and a trusting relationship with the patient.

WHY NOT THE NURSE ALSO?

Since there is no logical reason for confining this function to the physician, the responsibility for writing a DNR order and documenting the discussion with the patient in the progress notes should be, rather, a responsibility shared by the responsible physician and the responsible nurse, either the primary nurse or the head

---

Since there is apparently no logical reason for confining the responsibility for writing and documenting a DNR order to the physician, this responsibility should be shared by the responsible physician and the responsible nurse.

---

nurse, depending on the system of nursing care used. The writing of a DNR order should be regarded as an *overlapping function* of medicine and nursing, which may be performed by either the physician or the nurse depending on the situation. The idea that the nurse as well as the physician should be authorized to write DNR orders seems so eminently reasonable that one must wonder how the present arrangement endured so long.

In view of the roles of the nurse and the physician in relation to patients with terminal illnesses, and given the nonmedical nature of a DNR decision, it must be concluded that the function of writing a DNR order, once the decision is made by the patient or whoever makes the decision in the case of an incompetent patient, belongs at least as much to the role of the nurse as to the role of the physician.

The issue here is not professional interest in territoriality. It is how the patient will be best served. It is apparent from experience and from the literature that the long-standing problems that nursing has had in this regard have generally been rooted in the frequent failure of physicians to function responsibly in writing DNR orders. When this happens, the nurse is often put in a difficult position, and most importantly, the patient is not well served. *The interest of the patient will be best served if the responsible nurse, as well as the responsible physician, is authorized by the DNR policy of the hospital to write DNR orders.*

This argument is strengthened by the following considerations: First, it is often the nurse who initiates a discussion with the physician about the possibility of a DNR order because it is often the nurse, due to the frequent and ongoing interaction with the patient, to whom the patient will first make known the desire to have treatment cease and to be allowed to die. The nature of the nurse's role is such that these conversations often occur more naturally with the nurse than with the physician. In such situations, it makes good sense for the nurse, after consultation with the physician and other appropriate persons, to write the DNR order and its justification in the progress notes. The decision of the patient is more likely to be honored in this arrangement than if the nurse must communicate the patient's wish to the physician, who must then take up the matter with the patient and then write the order. Too frequently, physicians cannot be persuaded to discuss the question with the patient, and conversely, the patient has a notoriously difficult time discussing anything with the physician during the brief daily visit. This problem becomes more acute for the patient with terminal disease.

Second, regardless of who writes the DNR order, it is almost inevitably the nurse who carries it out by deliberate inaction. Because of the frequent failure of physicians to communicate with nurses about DNR orders that they write and to provide justification for the orders in the progress notes, nurses are sometimes confronted with DNR orders without any supporting information.

This dilemma is compounded because it is not unheard of for a physician to write a DNR order for a competent patient without discussing it with the patient. Thus, when there is a DNR order that has not been discussed with the nurse nor justified in the progress notes, the nurse can never be sure that the patient has consented to it. If the patient has cardiac arrest before the nurse has the opportunity to clarify the situation, what should be done? Should the order be honored in the hope that the patient has consented to it or should it be disregarded, running the risk of violating the patient's decision and incurring the physician's wrath? If nurses were authorized to write DNR orders, the incidence of such situations would be reduced and the probability that the patient's decision would be implemented without complication would be greatly increased.

Third, the authorization of the nurse to write DNR orders is consistent with the definition of nursing set forth by the American Nurses' Association (ANA) in its *social policy statement*, which defines nursing as "the diagnosis and treatment of human responses to actual or potential health problems."[13] Although this definition has its origin in the language of the 1972 Nurse Practice Act of New York State, its present widespread currency within the profession seems to be largely due to its incorporation in this official ANA document. The proposal that nurses as well as physicians be authorized to write DNR orders is consistent with the understanding of nursing embodied in this widely cited definition (C. Murphy, EdD, written communication, April 16, 1982).

The decision of the patient to refuse resuscitation efforts is a "human response" to terminal illness and the resultant, radically reduced quality of life. The "diagnosis" of that response as coherent and genuine and the "treatment" based on that diagnosis, ie, writing a DNR order and the corresponding documentation of the patient's decision in the progress notes, are clearly within the domain of nursing as defined by the ANA. Even so, how does the fact that this function falls within nursing's definition of itself support the argument that the patient is better served when the nurse is also authorized to write DNR orders? The broader argument is that patients will be better served if nurses are allowed to practice nursing within the scope of nursing without the constraints of medical authority.

The medical profession must be reassured by the enthusiastic support by the nursing profession of a definition of nursing that confines nursing's focus to the human response to disease and illness. But even this modest definition of nursing clearly encompasses the writing of DNR orders. Can the medical profession be anything but grateful for such a proposal, which promotes a definition of nursing that is so modest in its relation to medicine and proposes to relieve the profession of sole responsibility for such a burdensome task?

It can be suggested that only the physician is sufficiently responsible to carry the burden of such a grave act. It is the height of incongruity to suggest that the nurse, who must bear the life and death responsibility for initiating CPR when there is no DNR order, is somehow not sufficiently responsible to write a DNR order in the patient's chart once the patient has made the decision.

But perhaps nurses do not *want* this responsibility. This should not occasion any great surprise. Probably physicians have not wanted the responsibility either, which may be, in part, why they have carried it out so poorly. It is irrelevant whether nurses want the responsibility. What nurses want is not the basis of the argument. Patients would be better served if nurses shared the responsibility with physicians. In light of this and in light of the

---

It is incongruous to suggest that the nurse, who bears the life and death responsibility for starting CPR when there is no DNR order, is not sufficiently responsible to write the order once the patient has made the decision.

---

frustrations that nurses have experienced with physicians in regard to DNR orders, nurses will willingly assume the responsibility even though they may not "want" it.[12]

NOT FREE TO BE MORAL

Why should there be such a controversy over what may appear to be such a small matter? The answer is that this is one of several areas in patient care in which there are vestiges of the historical devaluation of the work of the nurse and violation of the autonomy of the nurse by physicians and hospitals, generally to the detriment of the patient. Ashley has eloquently documented the history of the oppression, exploitation, and devaluation of nurses by physicians and hospitals.[14] (This book should be required reading for every nursing student and perhaps, more importantly, for every medical student. A 4th-year medical student told us recently that he did not understand why nurses are so angry at physicians. We told him that his perplexity as a neophyte is understandable and recommended reading Ashley as a sure cure.)

The most recent witness to this reality is contained in the public hearing testimony before the National Commission on Nursing. Four of the five nursing problems most frequently mentioned corroborate Ashley's perception:
- the "status and image of nursing,"
- the "effective management of the nursing resource (staffing, scheduling, and salary),"
- the "relationship among nursing [staff] medical staff, and hospital administration,"

• and the "maturing of nursing as a self-determining profession."[15]

In its initial report, the Commission commented on "the fundamental unresolved nursing issues. One of the most fundamental of these is lack of recognition for nurses' worth in patient care."[16] One manifestation of this problem is the assignment of nursing responsibility in patient care without the authority necessary to fulfill that responsibility. The nurse is given a task that cannot be done without the pro forma cooperation of the physician; then it is often impossible to obtain the necessary cooperation. An excellent example is in the management of pain. Pain management is de facto a nursing function, regardless of its de jure status, but it cannot be performed without the pro forma cooperation of the physician, who sometimes does not order adequate medication and sometimes cannot be contacted when the order needs to be changed. The necessary authority is inappropriately vested solely with the physician. Because these kinds of situations abound in nursing practice, nurses have been aptly characterized as "the responsible powerless."[17]

In many situations involving DNR orders, pain management, or other aspects of patient care, Curtin's words are true: "Nurses are not free to practice nursing."[18]

The nurse in these situations is often not free to be moral, that is, a nurse is often not free to honor the commitment to the patient, whether that commitment takes the form of responding to the patient's request for no further treatment, of keeping the patient free from unnecessary suffering, or of performing whatever functions may be required by professional standards of nursing and by excellence in nursing practice.

The moral predicament of hospital nurses is that they often are not free to be moral because they often are not free, due to institutional contraints to exercise their commitment to the patient through excellence in patient care.

The fundamental moral predicament of hospital nurses is that they often are not free to be moral because they often are not free to exercise their commitment to the patient through excellence in patient care. Legal and institutional constraints hinder the practice of nursing sometimes in minor matters and sometimes in major matters of life and death. For the sake of patient care, the nurse must be set free to practice nursing, ie, set free to be moral.

There appears to be a growing consensus on this point among those concerned with nursing ethics. This concern found its way into the literature in 1978, for the first time, when Davis and Aroskar[19] asked the bold and fateful question, "Can the nurse be ethical?" The language is different from that of Curtin[18] in 1980, which was cited previously, but the point is the same. Most recently, in 1981, Mitchell argued that "nurses are unable to maintain their integrity."[8(p7)]

This analysis has implicit assumptions that need to be expressed. On the first level, the argument is that the interest of the patient is best served when the responsible nurse, as well as the responsible physician, is authorized to write DNR orders. The assumption here is that the interest of the patient lies in the preservation and actualization of patient autonomy. The policy objective is to serve the autonomy of the patient. Patient autonomy is honored when patients are effectively given final decision-making authority over their own care. Because the conditions of autonomy are often compromised by illness, special care must be taken to preserve patient autonomy. This is morally necessary because autonomy is the first principle of morality,[20] and it is psychologically important because patients, in the alien environment of the hospital, often experience a traumatic sense of loss of control and thereby a loss of social well-being as well as physical well-being.

Patients retain ultimate control over their own care insofar as those charged with that care involve them in significant decisions regarding their own care, provide them with all relevant information as a basis for decision making, enable them to reach decisions consistent with their considered and settled values, and then implement those decisions responsibly. The authorization of the responsible nurse, as well as the responsible physician, to write DNR orders will serve to promote the patient's autonomy in these ways. *If this argument holds, then the hospital is morally obligated to authorize the responsible nurse to write DNR orders.* If the preservation of the patient's autonomy is morally obligatory, then so is the best available means to that end. One cannot be obligated to the end without also being obligated to the best available means.

On the second level, the argument is that because of the historic domination of nursing by medical authoritarianism and repressive institutional policy, the nurse is often not free to be moral in the sense that she is often not free to exercise her professional commitment to the patient. The assumption here is that the patient will be best served if the nurse is empowered to actualize professional commitment to the patient. This assumption is not based on the further assumption that nurses are more virtuous than physicians or more committed to the well-being of the patient but rather on the assumption that the patient will be best served by a *balance of power around the bedside.* This precludes any one professional group from the unrestrained pursuit of its own interest at the expense of the patient. The presumed necessity for this balance of power rests on the same dim but realistic view of human nature that gave rise to the division and balance of power in government in democratic to protect the citizen against the tyranny of the state.

SOCIAL ETHICS AND INSTITUTIONAL REFORM

The business of setting the nurse free to practice nursing, ie, free to be moral, must proceed on various fronts. It is partly a matter of nurses achieving internal or psychological freedom after generations of socialization into a subordinate role both as nurses and women;[21] it is partly a matter of nurses acquiring the appropriate paradigm to understand the nature of health care and their role in it,[22] and it is partly a matter of institutional reform. It is the latter that is the concern of these reflections. The reform of the hospital as the major institutional context of and constraint on the practice of nursing is a matter of the utmost urgency from a moral perspective. Historically, nursing ethics has taken the form of individual ethics with a focus on the individual practitioner and the nurse–patient relationship. The time has come when an adequate nursing ethic must address the problem of the structures and policies of the institutions that constitute the context of nursing practice. A nursing ethic that addresses these kinds of concerns is a social ethic, ie, an ethic concerned with the moral obligations of institutions rather than with the moral obligations of individuals.

As the institutional context of practice more and more determines the nature and quality of the nurse–patient relationship and the quality of nursing care that is possible to provide, nursing ethics must become, in part, social ethics, addressing those institutional constraints that keep nurses from practicing nursing in accord with professional standards and the interest of the patient. This theme of the importance of social or institutional ethics has recently been quite pronounced in the medical ethics literature. Since the bureaucratization of medical care has become an acknowledged fact,[23] there is growing attention to the necessity for hospitals and institutions to assume appropriate responsibility for the moral dilemmas current in the practice of medicine. Hospitals are being challenged to consider themselves as moral agents with significant moral responsibilities.[24-26]

Various institutional reforms would contribute to setting nurses free from the constraints of medical authority and institutional policies. One reform that is often suggested is upgrading the status of nursing administration within the power structure of the hospital. This may be accomplished, at least in part, by moving the director of nursing service to a vice presidential level and adjusting the salary to a level commensurate with the salary of the chiefs of staff of the various medical services. These are important strategies in setting nursing free from medical authority in the hospital, but no less important is the kind of reform that directly affects the clinical practitioners of nursing rather than nursing administrators.

It is essential to formulate specific policies that will invest the clinical nurse with the authority to perform, without constraint, those responsibilities that, by their nature, belong to the role of the nurse, such as requesting psychiatric or social work consultation,[27] writing DNR orders, and the writing of pain medication orders. (The federal law limiting the distribution of regulated substances to physicians is a legal constraint impeding the responsible practice of nursing in the management of patients with pain and will require reform to free nurses to be fully responsible to their patients [C. Duffy, personal communication, April 16, 1982].) This type of reform must proceed clinical issue by clinical issue as nurses claim the authority that is necessary in specific types of clinical situations to responsibly fulfill their commitments to patients.

The liberation of nurses and their enfranchisement as moral agents and autonomous providers in the patient care enterprise need to be accomplished at the clinical as well as at the administrative level. Situations requiring DNR decisions have long been a source of conflict and frustration for the nurse because the nurse has been "the responsible powerless." Policies and laws that legitimate this state of affairs are without justification and must be viewed as a hindrance to excellence in patient care. They are in need of reform.

One obvious place to begin is with hospital DNR policy. Hospitals that have yet to establish such a policy should consider authorizing the responsible nurse as well as the responsible physician to write DNR orders. Hospitals that have already established policy only to find that it is frequently not honored by physicians should consider the proposed reform as a way to help resolve these ongoing problems. Hospitals, as institutions that constitute the context of practice for both medicine and nursing, have a moral obligation to establish policies that require those procedures most likely to serve the interest of the patient.

The DNR policy is a clear instance of the type of moral issue in nursing in which the resolution is dependent on the assumption of moral responsibility by the hospital. Nursing ethics, as social ethics, calls for the moral maturation of the hospital as a responsible social institution. Clinical nurses who practice in hospitals and are embroiled in these issues must make themselves heard, and nursing administration must provide them with firm support. The 1965 ANA position paper on nursing education[28] set the terms for freeing nursing *education* from the domination of medical authoritarianism and the hospital. It now remains to free nursing *practice* from this same debilitating domination, through the reform of institutional policy that regulates the relation of medicine to nursing and impedes the responsible practice of nursing. If nursing fails to free itself from this historical bondage to medical authoritarianism, it will fail the patient as well as itself. As Ashley[14] has shown it is not only power that corrupts, it is also powerlessness.

REFERENCES

1. Alder DC: No code—The unwritten order. *Heart and Lung* 1977;6(2):213.
2. Aroskar M, et al: The nurse and orders not to resuscitate. *Hastings Cent Rep* 1977;7(4):27-28.
3. Berg DL: The right to die dilemma. *RN* 1977; 40(7):1-7.
4. Cawley MA: Euthanasia: Should it be a choice? *Am J Nurs* 1977;77:859-861.
5. Johnson P: The long, hard dying of Joe Rodriques. *Am J Nurs* 1977;77:54-57.
6. Regan A: Nursing service problem: Verbal orders. *Regan Rep* 1977;17(10):4.
7. Steidl SN: Have you ever regretted doing the "right" thing? *RN* 1979;42(8):78D-78F.
8. Mitchell C: New directions in nursing ethics. *Massachusetts Nurse* 1981;50(7):7-10.
9. Curtin LL: The prostitution of CPR. *Supervisor Nurse* 1979;10(8):7.
10. Yarling RR: Ethical analysis of a nursing problem: The scope of nursing practice in disclosing the truth to terminal patients. *Supervisor Nurse* 1978;9(5):40-50 and 9(6):28-34.
11. Mill JS, Mill HT: *Essays on Sex Equality*, Rossi AS (ed). Chicago, University of Chicago, 1970, p 130.
12. Gewirth A: *Reason and Morality*. Chicago, University of Chicago, 1978, pp 49-52.
13. *Nursing—A Social Policy Statement*. Kansas City, Mo, American Nurses' Association, 1980, p 9.
14. Ashley JA: *Hospitals, Paternalism, and the Role of the Nurse*. New York, Teachers' College Press, Columbia University, 1976.
15. National Commission on Nursing: *Summary of Public Hearings*. Chicago, Hospital Research and Educational Trust, 1981, p 5.
16. National Commission on Nursing: *Initial Report and Preliminary Recommendations*. Chicago, Hospital Research and Educational Trust, 1981, p 10.
17. White AJ: Forum on DNR policy. University of Illinois College of Nursing, Mar, 1982.
18. Curtin L: Ethical issues in nursing practice and education, in *Ethical Issues in Nursing and Nursing Education*. New York, NLN, 1980, p 27.
19. Davis A, Aroskar M: *Ethical Dilemmas and Nursing Practice*. New York, Appleton-Century-Crofts, 1978, p 43.
20. Immanuel K: *Foundations of the Metaphysics of Morals*, Beck LW (trans). Indianapolis, Bobbs-Merrill, 1959, p 59.

21. Muff J (ed): *Socialization, Sexism, and Stereotyping: Women's Issues in Nursing*. St. Louis, CV Mosby, 1982.
22. Aroskar MA: Are nurses' mind sets compatible with ethical practice? *Top Clin Nurs* 1982;4(1):22-32.
23. Mechanic D: *The Growth of Bureaucratic Medicine*. New York, Wiley-Interscience, 1976.
24. Pellegrino ED: Hospitals as moral agents, in *Humanism and the Physician*. Knoxville, Tenn, University of Tennessee, 1979.
25. Pellegrino ED: The hippocratic oath revisited, in *Humanism and the Physician*. Knoxville, Tenn, University of Tennessee, 1979.
26. DeGeorge RT: The moral responsibility of the hospital. *J Med Philos* 1982;7(1):87-100.
27. Donnelly G: Anatomy of a conflict. *Supervisor Nurse* 1975;6(11):28-38.
28. American Nurses' Association: ANA's first position on education for nursing. *Am J Nurs* 1965;65(12):106-111.

The Nurse's Role in Protecting the Patient's Right to Live or Die

Elsie L. Bandman, R.N., Ed.D.
Associate Professor of Nursing
Bellevue School of Nursing
Hunter College
New York, New York

Bertram Bandman, Ph.D.
Professor of Philosophy
Brooklyn Center
Long Island University
Brooklyn, New York

SIGNIFICANCE OF THE PROBLEM FOR NURSES

LIFE IS REGARDED in western culture as one's "unalienable right" and codified in the words of the American "Declaration of Independence."

> We hold these truths to be self-evident, that all men are created equal, that they are endowed by their creator with certain unalienable rights, that among these are life, liberty, and the pursuit of happiness.[1]

These words underscore the concept of life as the prized possession of the individual necessary for freedom and for the pursuit of the conditions for individual and collective happiness. These principles, in their abstract form, are universally considered essential to the conditions of a just and moral society. Equality of opportunity and treatment is avidly sought by supporters of the Equal Rights Amendment, minorities and the American Nurses' Association in its support of the right of all to health care.[2]

On further examination, however, these principles called "truths" by our founding fathers are ineffective in major areas of contemporary life. One area of controversy is the individual's loss of the unalienable right to life, liberty and the pursuit of happiness in cases of national emergency such as war. The nation requires suspension of the individual's freedom on behalf of its prior right to defend itself against acts of perceived aggression. The individual's liberty, and possibly life, is sacrificed for the common welfare. Similarly, capital punishment is still practiced in some states on the basis of the community's right to punish by resorting to the ancient principle of "an eye for an eye, a tooth for a tooth" and of course a life for a life.

The most neglected but now controversial area of the application of the principle of the unalienable right to life may be in health care where issues of rights to live or die are critical and central for both care recipients and providers. The nursing care of the terminally ill, incurably disabled child and adult, as examples, raises complex issues of ethical decision and patient advocacy. Nurses are in the patient environment continuously with frequent opportunities for client and family contact with knowledge of their expressed wishes. How are nurses to use this knowledge on behalf of the patient? To whom are nurses accountable for their responses—the patient, themselves, the family, the physician, the hospital, the profession or society? How may nurses best protect the patient's right to live or die?

In caring for the incurably ill or hopelessly disabled person, nurses are traditionally placed in the position of double agents attempting to represent the interests

In caring for the incurably ill or hopelessly disabled person, nurses are traditionally placed in the position of double agents attempting to represent the interests of both the patient and the physician as the locus of authority.

of both the patient and the physician as the locus of authority. Nurses report that too often they are confronted with a lack of orders indicating how many times the patient should be resuscitated, if at all, or informed of the basis for the particular decision, including that of no decision. Annas reported that one 70-year-old woman was resuscitated over 70 times within a few days.[3] Nurses report that orders not to resuscitate are frequently written in pencil on the nurses' cardex and then destroyed on the patient's discharge. Verbal orders with double messages such as "make haste slowly" are said to be common. Moreover, physicians may leave orders which are contrary to the patient's and family's wishes either to continue the life of a beloved aged parent or to end the suffering of a cherished family member. The patient's wishes may be blatantly disregarded or, as in the case of the elderly woman, her best interests may be disregarded in the rigid adherence to the principle of continuing life.

Nurses often find themselves in the middle of conflicting viewpoints, such as those of the patient and of the family in opposition to the hierarchical medical establishment. Nurses may find their views difficult to advance because of lack of familiarity with an ethical or rights framework supportive of an analytical consideration of the differing views of a particular situation.

These are some of the issues which confront nurses as they participate in nursing care in an interdisciplinary matrix within an institutional context. The problems are numerous and complex. The vital missing ingredient for nursing participation in ethical decisions has been a theoretical framework which may serve as a reference point for decision making on a rational rather than an intuitive basis.

THE ROLE OF RIGHTS IN DECISION MAKING

Although some persons and groups use rights as expressions of powers in conflicts between persons and groups (such as conflicts between patients and health professionals, between physicians and nurses, between members of families or between interest groups and nation states), the concept of rights would be impoverished and fairly useless if rights did not have a role additional to that of expressing powers. What could this other role be?

Rights as generally conceived also have a role in settling disputes and in providing verdicts that are mutually acceptable to various parties, presumptively on rational grounds, grounds that either or any party would accept if their roles were reversed.

Rights may be defined as justifications for action. People who invoke a right can accordingly be understood to have a reason for acting. Individuals' rights to their own home or body, for example, justify their refusing others entry to their domain.

As we look at rights, however, we find that of the two commonly identified kinds of rights, option rights and welfare rights, these do not have much, if any, role in dispute settling, nor does there seem to be a way of justifying decisions in cases of conflict between these two kinds of rights.

Option Rights

Option rights mark a person's "sphere of autonomy," or freedom of action without interference by others. They include the right not to do what one has a right to do.

In history, this earliest kind of right has been associated with freedom. For Thomas Hobbes, a right meant the liberty to preserve one's existence; this right has come to be known as the right to self-preservation.[4(p84-85)] Some scholars even date these rights, sometimes referred to as "liberty-rights," to a medieval philosopher, William of Ockham, who defined a right as the use of a power in accordance with reason.[5(p48)] For John Locke, who followed Hobbes, rights also function as liberties toward self-preservation. Locke wrote his famous *The Second Treatise of Civil Government* shortly before "The Declaration of Independence" was written. Locke added that every person had a right to "life, liberty and estate."[6(p163,184)] "Estate" has been variously interpreted by some writers as one's property shares or holdings and by others as one's life and liberty.[7(p4-5)]

In our time, these option rights have been defended by a scholar such as Robert Nozick as vitally necessary "entitlements" for defending oneself against any oppressive state.[8(p150-182)]

These option rights, which certainly appeal to a morally powerful and important tradition, namely the desire for freedom, touch a vital mainspring in human nature. Far from being simply an ideal, the value of freedom manifests itself daily in the health professional's respect for the patient's autonomy and dignity. It is applied, for example, to such important values as privacy, confidentiality, the patient's right to give informed consent and to refuse treatment. We teach health care students to object to and disapprove of incidents such as the one in which Nurse Ratched, in *One Flew Over the Cuckoo's Nest*, tells the patient McMurphy to take his pill "because it's good for you."[9] To Nozick, individuals have a right to whatever they earn by work. For him, any form of taxation above and beyond that required for a police force and other essential public services needed to minimize homicide, theft and fraud is a reprehensible form of "forced labor."[8(p169)] For Nozick, rights provide individuals with a morally separate existence and the only justification for a state is to protect such individuals.

In medicine, Sade expresses the notion of rights as forms of freedom whereby a physician, a bricklayer, candlestick maker, baker, shoemaker or farmer can make a living.[10] For Sade, having a right means having the equal opportunity to pursue one's living without interference from others except to prevent harm to them.

Critics of option rights, however, regard them as forms of laissez faire morality, and contend that the exercise of these rights without limits can be and is harmful to others.

Welfare Rights

As a consequence of the lack of limits of these older option rights and of the unmet needs of large numbers of poor and powerless people, another kind of right emerged in the late 19th century. When the poor or helpless do not have enough of either food, shelter, education or health care, as illustrated for example in literature by the destitute orphan children in Dickens's *Oliver Twist*, they are in need of rights of another kind. These have been variously called rights of recipience[11] or assistance[12] or welfare rights.[13]

Welfare rights consist of the publicly supported distribution of food, clothing, shelter, education, health care, maternity benefits, social security and in some cases jobs to those in need. In some instances resources are provided to the public at large, such as publicly financed schools, museums, libraries, parks and public health services including safe water and vaccinations.

As option rights point to the highly honored value of freedom with its philosophical forbears in Locke and Kant, the welfare rights tradition appeals to another morally significant value, namely helping to alleviate human suffering and to maximize happiness.

The philosophical tradition that undergirds welfare rights stems primarily from the 19th century social philosophers, Jeremy Bentham and John Stuart Mill, who also did much to bring about child labor reform and other public welfare measures. The principle they appealed to was that of "the greatest happiness of the greatest number."[14(p10)] Their moral concern was to justify actions in proportion as they decreased the total suffering and pain felt by human beings and as they increased the total available pleasure. However, the pursuit of this goal, utilitarianism, is known to ignore the rights and dignity of individuals and minorities when these conflict with the happiness of the group.

The Conflicts of Rights

A point about both these rights is that while it does not seem possible for people in contemporary society to get along without some welfare rights, different economic groups of people seem to prize these rights differently. The poor prefer welfare rights and make claims for more rights of that kind, whereas the moderately well to do complain of having to pay more through increasing taxation for services they may not need. One conclusion about these kinds of rights is fairly certain. The older option rights which provide for the freedom of people to do what they can do for themselves unaided by others except to prevent unjustified interference, are less expensive than welfare rights, which require positive action by the state to provide publicly distributed resources. As a result, there is a growing conflict between the older and the newer rights, between option rights and welfare rights. To compound matters, there are also more and more aggravated conflicts between holders of option rights themselves (in, for example, mounting malpractice suits) and increasing conflicts of rights among recipients of welfare rights. As resources dwindle and populations and needs rise,

demands for more freedom and for even more welfare rights similarly escalate.

Consequently the language of rights, which began and was intended to serve as a means of justifying making morally defensible decisions for the distribution of freedom and the fair allocation of resources, has become so caught up in the conflicts of rights that rights are in danger of losing their traditionally important role in justifying decisions and action and in settling disputes. In this connection, Oliver Wendell Holmes once noted that the function of a judge in a dispute is to decide "who has gained the rights."[15(p21)] Rights in unending conflict become incapable of being appealed to in settling disputes or in justifying action. This means to a seriously ill patient who may wish to exercise the right to live or die and to the nurse who may feel obligated to protect the patient's rights, that these rights become inoperative as they are caught up in the maze of conflicting rights with few if any rights being honored.

Rights as a Basis for Settling Disputes

Some philosophers along with other notable scholars have recently argued that because rights now seem unserviceable, we may need to look for another moral and

---

Rights are and can be a rationally useful basis for settling disputes between right holders and for justifying decisions. In particular, rights are helpful to the nurse in protecting the patient's right to live or die.

political concept.⁵ However, rights are and can be a rationally useful basis for settling disputes between right holders and for justifying decisions. In particular, rights are helpful to the nurse in protecting the patient's right to live or die. Rights can be useful in settling disputes on criticisms that nurses would make about both option and welfare rights. Option rights without limits are socially irresponsible. The medical researcher may expose subjects to high risk with no benefit and without their knowledge. Tobacco growers and producers do not voluntarily stop their profitable but life-destroying activities. There are too few rationally effective restrictions against the harmful practices of option rights. The result of the insufficiently restricted growth of these option rights is that they rapidly erode into powers that do not justify action but that distribute more power to the powerful, thus giving rise to both more conflict and harm.

The scene for welfare rights fares no better. More and more claims and demands are made for goods and services that extend beyond available resources. The result is the *thinning out* of rights.¹⁶ For all cannot demand services when there are not enough to go around. Here too the result is not only aggravated conflict between different welfare rights, but the erosion of rights into powers, with little or no regard for the role of rights as rational dispute-settling devices and as justifications for action. Patients in circumstances where power and privilege replace rights cannot have their rights to live or die recognized and respected, especially if they are powerless to enforce their wishes.

A Third Right—The Legislative Right

While option and welfare rights are valuable and important, there is some basis in other social systems, historical and contemporary, to support a third right, one that offsets the difficulties of these earlier rights. Whereas the earlier rights are freedom based and happiness based, undoubtedly important values in any adequate account of moral values, these are not sufficient to provide for a defensible view of rights.

Those who turn to the ancient Greeks as well as to the Old Testament and Roman and Christian moral and political thought or to judicial systems in tribal societies appreciate that rights are based not only on freedom and happiness; rights are perhaps even more importantly based on justice. Possibly paraphrasing St. Augustine, some of his interpreters have held that there are no rights without justice. Neither the freedom nor happiness of some assures just settlement of disputes.

Both option rights and welfare rights may be regarded from an agent's view or from the social interplay of several agents' points of view as actors in a moral, political and legal context. There is another perspective, however, different from what the agent can do or receive in interaction with other agents, and that is the perspective not of a moral actor or agent but that of an evaluator, assessor-legislator or rule-maker, one who establishes (or a group of whom establish) the ground rules for deciding the justifiable extent and limits of both option rights and welfare rights. For without this more basic right, which may variously be called "the right to make rules" or the right to make law,[17(p53)] which we will call here legislative rights,[18] there would be no other kinds of operative rights at all, neither option (freedom) rights nor welfare (recipience) rights. For the determination of rules stipulating how much freedom and how much allocation individuals are entitled to receive in the form of welfare rights is logically, conceptually and historically prior to the attribution and exercise of option and welfare rights.

These legislative rights may be vested in a sovereign or a group and may take aristocratic, oligarchical or preferably democratic form. But no matter how these rights are exercised, no political society or set of option and welfare rights can exist without these prior legislative rights.

Legislative rights are not only prior; they also give significance to option and welfare rights and provide a means of settling disputes that occur when some claim more than their freedom or their share of benefits. One reason is that legislative rights, or rights viewed from the perspective of the rule-maker, to be appropriately operative, depend on another value, one which makes both freedom and happiness possible—that is justice.

Justice regulates the role of freedom and some conditions for achieving happiness. Justice provides for fair and equal freedom along with a fair and equal set of distributive shares. What fair and equal shares of freedom and conditions of happiness exactly amount to ought to be worked out by the members of a society.

Legislative rights consist of the right to participate in the governance and decision-making apparatus of one's community. Accordingly, such rights may also be referred to as "communal rights." These include not only the right to act as freely as possible with minimal interference and to receive as much assistance as possible (for everyone receives assistance at some time), but also the right to live significantly with others. That is why a democracy, theoretically as well as culturally and politically, is preferable to other forms. In a democracy, all people in principle have the right to participate equally in their community.

The right to legislate is not only fundamental and essential to any other kinds of rights, but is also vital to settling disputes and deciding cases (particularly euthanasia cases) in a just and rational manner.

One unargued assumption we make in presenting legislative rights is that rights do not occur outside a society. The right to freedom, for example, or the right to life is not derived from some source other than those who set the rules of a society. For option rights along with welfare rights depend on rules which mark out the extent and limits of freedom and welfare. Legislative rights provide that an individual's option rights and welfare rights are limited by the limits of a society's resources. Individuals who exercise legislative rights recognize that they and their fellow members are bound to live within the means of that society. These legislative rights are also limited by due process considerations and other moral proscriptions against majority or individual violation of rights. These rights are legislative in

> *Values that may be for the good of the majority at a given time may not be good for the long-term moral and political goals of that society.*

a prelegal moral sense analogous to the "Declaration of Independence," the "Preamble to the U.S. Constitution," sometimes referred to as the "Welfare Clause," and to the Bill of Rights.[18-20] Values that may be for the good of the majority at a given time may not be good for the long-term moral and political goals of that society. The economic circumstances of a community may make it advisable to restrict individual option rights, such as the right to produce harmful commodities or to continue to live or reproduce, if one is unable to fulfill functions needed by the society. A person who is comatose and brain dead may have an option right to live, but not a legislative right.

Legislative rights perform four roles, one initially in rule making,[17] a second in rule changing,[17] a third in moral constraints against unjust rules and a fourth in adjudication or dispute settling.[21]

The right to legislate is bound by the principle of universalization of similar cases; it cannot be the arbitrary right of a person or group to make rules inapplicable to an entire class of cases; for that is what the right to make rules means. Background principles of equal justice restrict the right to rule. As rules are equally binding with equal cases, rights governing the relation between freedom and welfare are justified, in turn, only if they rationally resolve disputes and allay conflicts which threaten a community.

CASES ILLUSTRATING DIFFERENT KINDS OF RIGHTS

The following cases illustrate how rights may have a decision-making role in the patient–nurse relationship. The more kinds of rights which can be appealed to in a given case, the stronger the rational basis for decision.

Case 1[22]

Mr. M was an unmarried 82-year-old resident of a nursing home independent in self care, and able to ambulate with a walker, but needing assistance in dressing. Despite occasional episodes of memory loss and confusion, he continued to care for himself. His loss of hearing interfered with social activities but he resisted the use of a hearing aid. The development of dysuria led to the diagnosis of benign prostatic hypertrophy and the recommendation of a trans-urethral prostatectomy. When informed of the necessity for surgery, Mr. M readily consented. His nephew and only relative, however, refused to consent to surgery on the grounds that because of his uncle's mental state, his life was without dignity and should not be sustained by extraordinary means. The nephew believed that the uncle had already lived a long life. The nurse verified the uncle's understanding and consent to the surgery to no avail. Without the surgery, Mr. M's condition rapidly declined and he died of uremic complications within six weeks.

Case 2

Schowalter, Ferholt and Mann[23] report the case of 16-year-old Karen who was Catholic and the second of seven siblings. She was hospitalized in 1968 for chronic, active glomerulonephritis. After two years of extensive treatment proved unsuccessful, both kidneys were removed. A transplant of her father's kidney was unsuccessful. Hemodialysis was performed prior to and following surgery. It caused her to have "chills, nausea, vomiting, severe headaches and weakness."[23(p97)] In April 1970, before the transplant, a child psychiatrist evaluated the family. Karen was viewed as having an appropriate reactive depression. The father immersed himself in professional activities. The mother was suspicious of the medical management, and evidenced "circumferential speech, loosening of thought associations, and an inappropriate lability of affect."[23(p97)] She was recommended for outpatient psychiatric treatment but this was not accomplished. Beginning in July 1970 "Karen and her parents met regularly"[23(p97)] with the child psychiatrist and a social worker prior to and following the transplant.

In April 1971 it became evident that the transplanted kidney would not function. "Karen and her parents expressed the desire to stop medical treatment."[23(p98)] The medical staff, however, found this decision unacceptable, and the psychiatrist and social worker tried to guide the family to reconsider their refusal of further medical care. The family agreed to continue Karen's hemodialysis, medication and prescribed diet at home. Karen's life

became one of isolation and restriction, with persistent discomfort and fatigue. The decision to resume treatment was rapidly followed by hospitalization for high fever and subsequent removal of the transplant. The shunt became infected, necessitating revision of both the shunt and the vein wall. On May 24, 1971, the shunt clotted and closed.

Thereupon, with her parents' consent, Karen refused further dialysis and shunt revision. The staff was frustrated and angry, believing this decision immoral, unsound and inappropriate for her age of 16 years. Karen discussed her decision with the hospital chaplain. She concluded that there was no hell and possibly no heaven, but that "nothingness would be far better than the suffering which would continue if she lived."[23(p98)]

The child psychiatrist "found no evidence of psychosis"[23(p98)] but rather a carefully considered, rational decision. Both the psychiatrist and the nephrologist decided that Karen's decision was rational and that the staff's duty was to comply by making her remaining life comfortable with daily counseling in the event she changed her mind. The staff considered such alternatives as requesting the court to force treatment or the parents to take Karen home to die so as to avoid staff assistance to an act of suicide. One nurse from the dialysis unit visited Karen and insisted that she return for further dialysis. Staff members who had witnessed Karen's prolonged suffering were more supportive of her decision.

Following her decision, Karen's spirits and appetite improved. She thanked the staff for their activities on her behalf, picked a burial place near her home, wished her parents happiness and supported them through the final days of her life and of their doubt regarding the decision. On June 2, 1971, she died suddenly and peacefully with both parents at her bedside.

Case 3

Ms. Brown, the mother of four young children, was abandoned by her husband when she became seriously ill following surgery in which cancer with metastasis was found in her pelvic region. She was given radiation treatment and is now on chemotherapy as the only hope for remission and prolongation of life. The side effects are decidedly unpleasant; nevertheless, with the aid of a housekeeper, visiting nurses, and a social worker provided by a home-care service, she is able to be at home with her children. She has been and continues to be a devoted mother, doing her utmost to provide loving parenting, guidance and wisdom to her children. In the event of her death, the children, ages three, six, eight and ten, will become charges of the state, there being no relatives able or willing to take over their care. The husband's whereabouts are unknown.

Despite her deep concern for the children and full knowledge that they will probably be separated after her death, and placed in foster homes, Ms. Brown wishes to end the daily bouts of retching, vomiting and malaise which the medication causes her. She wishes to hasten what she considers to be an inevitable death. Her nurses, physicians and social workers argue that such a decision would deprive the children of a loving, though often bedridden mother, a home and a family unit. In their view, each day that Ms. Brown is alive and at home is another day in which the children become more self-reliant in caring for themselves and each other in school, at home and at play.

Case 4

Myra Levine[24] reports the case of a dear friend who developed serious symptoms requiring an exploratory craniotomy, but who faced surgery with serenity. An inoperable widespread tumor was found and she was transferred to the intensive care unit in a deep coma. The neurosurgeon explicitly ordered that in the event of respiratory failure, no extraordinary measures were to be used. When her respiration ceased a few hours later, a nurse immediately began to administer oxygen by a face mask. Despite the family's pleas to the contrary, the physician believed that he could not then discontinue respiratory support for the next four days. At the time, the kidneys which the patient had wished to be donated "as a gift of life" and as the "one last gesture that she so fervently desired"[24(p843–849)] were useless.

APPLICATION OF THREE KINDS OF RIGHTS TO OUR CASES

In the first case, involving Mr. M, we find Mr. M's right to life in conflict with his nephew's right not to have to support his uncle. Clearly, the cost of supporting the uncle is a burden on the nephew, whether taken on by the nephew or by society. Someone other than the benefactor of the prostatectomy has to pay.

First, however, what about the nephew's claim that the uncle had lived long enough? Can such a claim on behalf of another be sustained? It does not seem that the nephew is really looking out for the best interests of his uncle. In a conflict between the nephew's rights and the uncle's option right to live, the uncle's right clearly overrides the nephew's inconvenience. But what if the cost of the operation places a burden on the nephew? The fact that the nephew is or feels burdened raises the question: Why is there no operative welfare right for Mr. M, one that would alleviate the burden of decid-

---

Our moral intuitions seem to strongly favor a person's right to live over the right of others to decide for another person that his life is not worth continuing.

---

ing whether a person has a right to live or die on the basis of expense?

Our moral intuitions seem, at least in this type of case, to strongly favor a person's right to live over the right of others to decide for another person that his life is not worth continuing, even though surgery and postsurgical support may be expensive. In this case, we contend that the uncle has a clear option right to live and be supported by means of his welfare rights and through legislative rights which appeal to rules developed for cases in this category.

In a just society, if he were in a position to do so, Mr. M's legislative rights would have entitled him to participate in making

the rules which would have granted him and others like him the right to have the vital surgery without consideration of cost as a function of his welfare rights. Mr. M's legislative rights would provide rules limiting everyone's option rights (to pay fewer taxes for example) in order to save the lives of those who need medical assistance.

One might argue that legislative rights might run the other way. But this confuses what a given majority would do as a short-sighted measure with what it ought to do as a matter of social justice to everyone. Thus the right to make rules for everyone would not permit the legislative right to place the cost of an operation ahead of a person's life, unless the community is under threat of extinction. Because of the moral restrictions governing the right to make rules for everyone, it can ordinarily not be a legislative right to make a rule placing the cost of an operation ahead of a person's right to life. If, however, the community is in peril either through extreme scarcity of basic resources or is under attack, the economic circumstances of the community may conceivably alter the legislative right Mr. M and everyone like him has to be cared for. But in our case, there seems to be no similar emergency which could justify depriving Mr. M of a needed prostatectomy on grounds of cost. In this case, therefore, all three kinds of rights support Mr. M's right to needed surgery.

In the second case, did 16-year-old Karen have a right to die? Since the right to live, as with any right, includes the right not to do what one has a right to do, Karen, having an option right to live, also has the right not to live.[25] In this type of case it seems that the welfare of others (such as dependent relatives or other members of the community) does not conflict with her right to die. To use a term of Ronald Dworkin's, we may say that Karen has a right to die because there are no "competing rights" that conflict with her right to die.

Her well-being seems to be the only consideration, one that a community cannot provide for except to enable her to exercise her right to die, since all attempts to treat her were unsuccessful.

The prior legislative right to make rules for similar cases clearly seems to favor Karen's right to die. Even St. Thomas Aquinas's argument, that "life is a gift"[26(p24)] that can be taken only by the giver of all gifts and not by anyone who is given the gift of life, seems to be a right that is too difficult to defend if the person who has life feels it is no longer a gift.

It seems clear therefore that Karen has a right to die, one that has no overriding welfare considerations which conflict with her right and one which a reasonable interpretation of a right to legislate would favor as a policy for similar cases.

The case of Ms. Brown is different. She has a right to die, but here there are the competing welfare rights of her children who need her. Ms. Brown's right to die is in conflict with her four children's rights to be taken care of and given at least one parent for as long as possible.

Even if the state could provide, it would not do so in this case as well as even a seriously sick mother. The work of Bowlby[27] on parental deprivation is relevant in weighing Ms. Brown's right to die against her four children's rights to have a mother

as long as possible. Unless there are surrogate parents, we think Ms. Brown's right to die is limited by the needs of her children.

But this type of case also reveals the need for more ample welfare provisions on behalf of replacement parenting when that seems indicated. After all, Ms. Brown will die fairly soon and this will leave four children with insufficient attention to their rights to develop and grow up to live decent and fulfilling human lives. Provisions for such welfare rights of otherwise orphaned children are made by initially established legislative rights.

A more humane and just society, one where the right to make fair and equal rules prevailed, would enable other surrogate mothers to take the burden off Ms. Brown, who lives only by suffering extreme pain and discomfort.

This case shows the importance not only of welfare rights, both of the mother and her children, but also the need for legislative rights which provide for welfare rights along with option rights. This case also shows that Ms. Brown's option right to die could have been honored had she lived in a society where others would readily regard her children as their children as well. But this honoring of her option rights could only come about in a society that gave prior recognition to the legislative rights to have ample provision for option rights along with welfare rights, making it unnecessary to regard any children whose natural parents were deceased as "orphans," especially with the emotional overtones that accompany the desperation that attends orphanhood in our society.

In this case as it is presented, it can be

reluctantly concluded that with this society's less than ample provision for the care of children, Ms. Brown's right to die clashes with the "competing right" of her children to parenting by her. Therefore the nurse's role is to protect the Brown children's rights to their mother as long as it is possible to keep her alive.

But our conclusion reveals only the lack of justice in our society and the absence of a just right to make rules. For if there were normative legislative rights, they would make provision for the Brown children's welfare rights, which in turn would enable Ms. Brown to exercise her option right to die.

In Case 4, we'll begin by calling the lady in Myra Levine's paper Ms. Green. Ms. Green, seriously ill, has requested that her kidneys be donated to someone in need. The MD orders no resuscitation in case of respiratory failure.

The nurse, however, exercises his/her option right of supplying oxygen when Ms. Green goes into respiratory failure. The nurse presumably believes in the right to life at all cost or at least is so habituated as to be unrestrained by the MD's orders not to resuscitate. The result is that after four days of intensive life-saving efforts by other physicians as well, Ms. Green dies, leaving her kidneys in an unusable condition.

In this case Ms. Green's option right not to be revived (if we may infer that as her wish) coincided not only with the welfare rights of potential recipients of her kidneys, but also with the moral basis of legislative rights designed to serve the good of the community. In this case then, the nurse's option right of deciding to save Ms. Green's life would conflict with Ms.

Green's option right to decide what happens in and to her body along with the welfare rights of a potential beneficiary together with the legislative right designed to promote the common good. In that case, therefore, the option, welfare and legislative rights that collided with the nurses's rights would provide a basis for deciding in favor of protecting the patient's wishes to end life.

PROTECTION MEASURES

By studying the three kinds of rights and their application to difficult cases, nurses can move ethical decisions from an intuitive to a rational and moral base. The most forceful elements in these three kinds of rights for nursing lie in their universal appeal to justice. These views of rights are applicable to all cases in which the patient's right to live or die is at issue and serve as justification for decision.

Although the nursing and medical staff involved in Karen's care in Case 2 were rendered helpless and angry by her decision to die, clearly there were no overriding rights to her option right to decide to die. Prolonging her suffering clearly was an injustice to her in these circumstances. In Case 3, there were overriding views of rights in opposition to the patient's expressed wish to die. These were the rights of her children and of the community to maintain an intact family for as long as possible to provide for the psychological, sociological and developmental needs of the young children for a nurturing figure and membership in a nuclear family unit. The options for these children were bleak.

In Case 4, all three kinds of rights

It is imperative that organized nursing find its voice and press for implementation of measures to protect the rights of patients to live or die.

support the patient's decision to die. No one, including herself, would benefit from her comatose state, but advantages accrued to the community in terms of conserving scarce resources, and to the individuals who received her kidneys as well as benefit to herself by way of a sense of continuing life in another human being. The nurse had no right to impose her own moral views in disregard of the patient's expressed wishes. In Case 1, the elderly person's right to life-saving surgery which he desired should have been supported by welfare rights and legislative rights. This decision based on its support by all three

kinds of rights would have been a rational one to be implemented by a just society.

Based on these views of rights, it is imperative that organized nursing find its voice and on the rational grounds presented press for implementation of measures to protect the rights of patients to live or die. This is sometimes accomplished at the informal level on a face-to-face basis in the nursing unit. However, it needs to be done formally, rationally and openly at the level at which the patient's wishes, the family's wishes, medical considerations of feasibility and prognosis, and universal principles of justice such as fairness are considered. A Bowery derelict's right to life is equal to a banker's right to life in a just society if both need a transurethral prostatectomy to survive, even though one is a financial burden to the community and the other is a benefactor.

REFERENCES

1. Second Continental Congress. *Declaration of Independence* (Philadelphia: Second Continental Congress, July 4, 1776).
2. American Nurses' Association. *The Right to Health Care* (Kansas City, Mo.: ANA 1978).
3. Annas, G. "Remarks on the Law-Medicine Relation: A Philosophical Critique." Trans-Disciplinary Symposium, on Philosophy and Medicine, Department of Community Medicine and Health Care, University of Connecticut Health Center, Farmington, Connecticut, November 11, 1978.
4. Hobbes, T. *Leviathan* (Oxford: Basil Blackwell 1928).
5. Golding, M. "Rights: A Historical Sketch" in Bandman, E. and Bandman, B., eds. *Bioethics and Human Rights: A Reader for Health Professionals* (Boston: Little, Brown and Co. 1978).
6. Locke, J. *Two Treatises of Government* (New York: Hafner Publishing Co. 1947).
7. Melden, A. I. "Introduction" in Melden, A. I., ed. *Human Rights* (Belmont, Calif.: Wadsworth Publishing Co. 1970).
8. Nozick, R. *Anarchy, State and Utopia* (New York: Basic Books 1974).
9. Kesey, K. *One Flew Over the Cuckoo's Nest* (New York: The Viking Press 1970).
10. Sade, R. M. "Medical Care as a Right: A Refutation." *N Engl J Med* 285:23 (December 2, 1971).
11. Raphael, D. D. "Human Rights: Old and New" in Raphael, D. D., ed. *Political Theory and the Rights of Man* (Bloomington, Ind.: Indiana University Press 1967) p. 54–67.
12. Olson, R. G. *Ethics: A Short Introduction* (New York: Random House 1978) p. 66–67.
13. Golding, M. "Towards a Theory of Human Rights." *Monist* 52:4 (October 1968) p. 521–549.
14. Mill, J. S. *Utilitarianism* (New York: Liberal Arts Press 1957).
15. Holmes, O. W. "The Path of the Law" in Kent, E. A., ed. *Law and Philosophy* (New York: Appleton-Century-Crofts 1971).
16. Bandman, B. and Bandman, E. "General Introduction" in Bandman and Bandman, eds. *Bioethics and Human Rights: A Reader for Health Professionals.*

17. Hart, H. L. A; *The Concept of Law* (Oxford: Clarendon Press 1961).

18. Dworkin, R. *Taking Rights Seriously* (Cambridge: Harvard University Press 1977) p. xii, xiii, 93, 105, 150–222.

19. Rawls, J. *A Theory of Justice* (Cambridge, Mass.: Harvard University Press 1971) p. 213, 133–136, 235–241.

20. MacCormick, D. N. "Rights in Legislation" in Hacker, P. and Raz, F., eds. *Law, Morality and Society: Essays in Honor of H. L. A. Hart* (Oxford: Clarendon Press 1977).

21. Golding, M. *The Philosophy of Law* (Fair Lawn, N.J.: Prentice-Hall 1975). p. 106–125.

22. "Gerontological Nursing Situation." Presented at the Conference Group's Program "Bucking the System," December 9, 1975. The New York Counties Registered Nurses Association, Inc., District 13 of the New York State Nurses Association, New York, New York.

23. Schowalter, J. E. et al. "The Adolescent Patient's Decision to Die." *Pediatrics* 51:1 (January 1973) p. 97–103.

24. Levine, M. "Nursing Ethics and the Ethical Nurse." *Am J Nursing* 77:5 (May 1977) p. 843–849.

25. Dempsey, D. *The Way We Die* (New York: McGraw-Hill Book Co. 1975) p. 110.

26. St. Thomas Aquinas. "The Sin of Suicide " in Abelson, R. and Friquegnon, M., eds. *Ethics for Modern Life* (New York: St. Martin's Press 1975).

27. Bowlby, J. *Attachment and Loss* Vol. I (New York: Basic Books 1969).

In Vitro Fertilization: Dilemma or Opportunity?

Ora L. Strickland, R.N., Ph.D.,
F.A.A.N
Associate Professor
University of Maryland
School of Nursing
Baltimore, Maryland

ON JULY 25, 1978, Lesley and Gilbert Brown celebrated the birth of their first child, Louise, at Oldham District General Hospital near London. This was not just an ordinary birth: Louise Brown was the first known "test-tube baby."

Louise Brown's birth represented an important scientific breakthrough. Drs. Steptoe and Edwards had previously reported reimplantation of a human embryo with a subsequent tubal pregnancy after in vitro fertilization,[1] so this birth did not surprise many in the scientific community. Although the procedure appeared relatively simple, it had taken years of research before it was successful.[1-5] Louise Brown's birth represented a long-awaited advancement in scientific technology, but at the same time it raised many questions and rekindled controversy about the moral, ethical, and legal implications of in vitro fertilization. Is such a technological feat necessarily a step forward? How will it affect some of the basic values that influence sexuality, the family, and parenthood? How might this technology affect the status and lives of women in society? This article will review some of the potential benefits and ethical, social, moral, and legal questions raised by human in vitro fertilization.

CLINICAL APPLICATIONS OF IN VITRO FERTILIZATION

Clinical in vitro fertilization research is conducted for the primary purpose of initiating a pregnancy and producing a child after in vitro fertilization. In vitro fertilization involves externalizing oocytes (mature eggs) and sperm prior to fertilization. It is a technological step beyond artificial insemination, which externalizes only sperm.

After oocytes have been stimulated to mature by the administration of human gonadotrophin, they are removed from their follicles before ovulation by a surgical method involving laparoscopy. As many as four preovulatory oocytes can be retrieved. The oocytes and sperm are brought into contact in a special medium, and fertilization occurs with a fraction of these eggs. The fertilized oocytes (zygotes) are subsequently placed in a prepared medium and observed for cleavage. After it has developed to the blastocyst stage, the embryo is reintroduced into the uterus through the cervix approximately 4 days after fertilization. In the next few weeks the woman's sex hormones are closely monitored for signs of implantation and pregnancy.[1,6] If all goes well, the gravid woman experiences a normal pregnancy and delivers a healthy newborn.

Is the technology of human in vitro fertilization a needed step forward? The desire to have children must be among the most basic of human instincts, but many couples are unable to bear their own children because of infertility problems. Tubal occlusion is among the leading causes of infertility. The extent of infertility due to tubal occlusion is unknown, but it has been estimated that infertility is a problem for 1 out of 10 married couples in the United States and that tubal factors account for approximately 32% of infertility problems.[7] A most immediate clinical application of in vitro fertilization is to aid in the impregnation of women who have a blockage in the fallopian tubes. Women who have been infertile because of tubal problems "could thereby have their own children, fathered by their own husbands."[8(p87)] It is possible that there will be a demand for thousands of babies by this means each year. The current need for the procedure also may be increased by women who decide to have children after voluntary sterilization by tubal ligation.[9]

In vitro fertilization versus reconstruction

Even though the benefit of in vitro fertilization for treating infertile women is readily recognized, several ethicists have reservations about this use of the procedure. Is it a basic right to have your own biological child at any expense? Should infertility be treated by any and all available means? Is it fiscally wise to treat infertility due to occlusion of the fallopian tubes by in vitro fertilization when reconstruction of the fallopian tubes might be the most sensible and cost-effective method for overcoming tubal obstruction? Such reconstruction "treats the

> *It seems wiser to direct efforts toward preventing one of the major causes of infertility rather than investing . . . money in developing clinical programs for providing in vitro fertilization.*

underlying disease, not merely the desire to have a child."[10(p26)] Ramsey noted that "if infertility is a 'clinical defect' [that] should be remedied, that would seem to call for reconstructive surgery on the oviducts, from which 30% to 50% success has been reported."[11(p148)] The estimated cost of a baby provided by in vitro fertilization is $5,000 to $10,000. This could greatly increase the health care bill in the United States. For an estimated 500,000 women with blocked fallopian tubes, the only hope of conceiving a child is through in vitro fertilization and embryo transfer.[12] Kass, a biologist and physician, pointed out that because the majority of women with blocked oviducts are infertile owing to gonorrhea and pelvic inflammatory disease, it would seem impractical to have a "program of 'petri-dish babies' before we had a vaccine against gonococcus."[12(p7),13(p55)] It seems much wiser to direct efforts toward preventing one of the major causes of infertility rather than investing large sums of money in developing clinical programs for providing in vitro fertilization.

In vitro fertilization and abortion

Hellegars and McCormick question the morality of clinical in vitro fertilization. They find it ironic that in a society where 1.3 million legal abortions are performed each year—mostly on healthy babies—the United States would substantially fund life-creating technologies. Once this practice begins, it may prove difficult to deny such services to women who cannot afford them and who are eligible for Medicaid. In vitro fertilizations for the treatment of infertility could become another expensive tax burden for the American taxpayer.[14]

Proponents of in vitro fertilization present an alternative view. They emphasize that infertility is a clinical defect that should be remedied, if possible, by medical attention. Edwards and Sharpe argue that the right of some couples to have children cannot be denied on ethical or other grounds and that the parents' physical health does not demand that their infertility be cured. Because it is no longer certain that children will be available for adoption as abortion becomes more acceptable, this emphasizes the need for in vitro fertilization for treating infertility.[8]

The use of in vitro fertilization as a means to relieve infertility has raised concern about two important ethical issues related to the procedure. First, some ethicists believe that relieving infertility through in vitro fertilization is morally impermissible because the procedure may incur a greater risk of spontaneous abortion of the implanted embryo or produce defective children.[6,10,15]

The second argument against clinical in vitro fertilization is that extra-utero conception is unnatural[10,11] and might result in total artificial manipulation of reproduction with dehumanized hatcheries similar to those described in Huxley's *Brave New World*.[16] Because approximately 45% of eggs that are fertilized as a consequence of sexual intercourse either do not successfully implant or go to term,[13,17] this weakens arguments regarding the morality of subsequent spontaneous abortion after in vitro fertilization and embryo transfer. If a person believes that abortion is not wrong or that women should have the right to abort an unwanted child, then an increased risk of spontaneous or induced abortion from in vitro conception techniques should not be sufficient reason for limiting the use of in vitro fertilization for reproductive purposes.[18]

A question of 'experimentation'

Ramsey views in vitro fertilization as unethical, not only because of the possibility of the increased potential for abortion but because it can be considered as experimentation on unconsenting "possible future human beings" for which the extent of possible harm from the procedure is not known.[15(p1346)] He believes that there has not been enough research with animals to perfect the procedure enough for it to be considered safe for procreating a human infant. However, Lappé notes that parents at risk for serious genetic defects in their offspring are not prohibited from procreating. Nor are other treatments for infertility discouraged, such as ovulation-induction hormonal treatments. These treatments carry risks of multiple births and the resultant risk of prematurity, which may be harmful to the offspring.[17] On the basis of this argument, society is unlikely to restrict in vitro fertilization because of possible defects to the unborn child unless substantial evidence indicates a risk to the child.

It will take years of research and possibly thousands of "test-tube babies" to determine the immediate and long-term effects of in vitro fertilization on the child procreated in such a manner.

The argument that clinical in vitro fertilization will lead to a large number of deformed babies seems unjustified. Any zygote that was significantly damaged would be unlikely to be carried to term in the first place, because most damaged zygotes either do not implant or are spontaneously aborted.[19] In reality it will take years of research and possibly hundreds, if not thousands, of "test-tube babies" to determine the immediate and long-term effects of in vitro fertilization on the child procreated in such a manner.

Unnatural aspects of in vitro fertilization

The issue of the unnaturalness of clinical in vitro fertilization has been raised primarily by Kass and Ramsey.[10,11] In vitro fertilization is viewed as an inhuman "transfer of procreation from the home to the laboratory.[10(p48)] Some people are concerned that human procreation will be transformed into reproduction through manufacturing progeny artificially in laboratories supplied with sperm and egg banks. It is feared that laboratory reproduction could therefore interfere with the union between sex, and love, and procreation. Kass warns that "to lay one's hands on human generation is to take a major step toward making man himself simply another one of the man-made things."[10(p49)]

Proponents of clinical in vitro fertilization research envision that another potential benefit of the procedure may be the reduction of the incidence of genetic defects through genetic engineering. Modification of the genetic constitution of the genetically defective embryo or adding to the embryo itself may be implemented prior to implantation to produce a healthy child. The possibility of cleaving human embryos in culture after in vitro fertilization provides an opportunity to interfere with development, particularly because only a few cells—perhaps only one— would need to be altered for the effects to be exerted in the resulting fetuses.[8,20] This also enlarges the possibility of predetermining the sex of offspring by reimplanting sexed embryos. Sexing could be eugenically beneficial because many genetic disorders are sex linked and usually occur in males. Chromosome examination and gene transfer also may prevent the birth of children with genetic anomalies such as mongolism.

The benefits of clinical in vitro fertilization research for the purpose of reducing birth defects are obvious. However, this technology raises opposition because it provides the means whereby elective sex determination and genetic selection may become widely practiced. Cloning and the generation of man-animal hybrids or "chimeras" also may be developed.

Potential for demographic imbalance

A major issue arising regarding sex determination is the potential for the undesirable side effect of a demographic imbalance between the sexes. Because most sex-linked genetic diseases occur in males, there could be an increase in the number of females compared with the number of males if sex predetermination is practiced for purely eugenic reasons. Edwards and Sharpe predict that the selection of females for eugenic reasons would take a long time to build into statistically significant proportions, if ever.[8] Many couples would be deterred by the effort required in this procedure, particularly when the same end could be achieved by selective abortion.[20] But what if parents are given the opportunity to use in vitro fertilization to choose male or female children? Could this result in a population with males highly outnumbering females? The concerns raised by such an imbalance suggest that an increase in male children could result in an increase in prostitution and homosexuality.[21] It is feared that even a small shift to an excess of males could lead to the "raiding" of younger age groups of women by older men.[8]

Ramsey views sex predetermination through in vitro fertilization as a type of genetic selection. The potential for genetic selection not only could lead physicians to comply with parents' desires to have a child of a particular sex but also to comply with such frivolous wishes as having a child with "blond hair rather than brown, or a genius rather than a clout."[11(p1481)]

Jones and Bodmer warn that the selective elimination of even defective genes from the population is so formidable that it must be done cautiously. Society should be reasonably certain that genetic selection is for the good of the person directly involved and for the good of society in general. The human race could be drastically altered if genetic selection is vigorously applied.[22]

Cloning

The potential for human cloning through a combination of in vitro fertilization, genetic engineering, and embryo transfer to the uterus for gestation and birth has led to outspoken remarks against clinical applications of in vitro fertilization. Cloning is a form of asexual reproduction whereby the nucleus can be removed from the ovum, replaced with the nucleus of a cell from a donor, and embryonic development initiated. The embryo could then be transferred into the uterus to grow, resulting in an exact genetic copy of the cell donor.[8,23]

Cloning of humans would raise several ethical and moral issues itself because the cloned offspring would know that he or she had the same genetic potential as a preceding individual. The development of clones to serve as organ donors for each other for transplants and the cloning of outstanding or specialized individuals to fulfill unique roles, as suggested by Fletcher, could have far-reaching societal implications.[24]

Concern that human-animal hybrids or "chimeras" may be an outcome of clinical in vitro fertilization assumes that it will be possible to successfully support the development of man-animal hybrids beyond the stage of viability. Fletcher suggests that such organisms might be useful to society to perform unrewarding, dull, or dangerous roles required for social welfare, although he indicates that "man-machine hybrids" would be preferable.[24(p83)] As with cloning, the development of chimeras

through the application of the technology of in vitro fertilization would undoubtedly place tremendous moral, ethical, and legal burdens on society. The ramifications would be grave.

LABORATORY IN VITRO FERTILIZATION RESEARCH

Some human in vitro fertilization embryos are grown and experimented on in the laboratory without any attempt to transfer them to the uterus for gestation and delivery. Laboratory research on fertilized human eggs is conducted for several reasons. This research promises an increased understanding of fertilization, implantation, and embryonic development of critical organ systems. Studies on human embryonic development could increase knowledge needed to help prevent congenital malformations and some highly malignant tumors, such as hydatidiform mole, which originate from aberrant fetal tissue. New birth control measures could be developed, based on new knowledge obtained from laboratory in vitro fertilization research.[12,13]

Morality of laboratory research

There are serious challenges regarding the morality of conducting human in vitro fertilization in the scientific laboratory for purely research purposes, particularly when the practice entails their sacrifice in the course of investigation. Two issues that have received the most discussion regarding the morality of laboratory in vitro fertilization are the moral status or "humanness" of the early embryo in the context of laboratory research and the need for informed consent from the donors of gametes prior to in vitro fertilization for research manipulation.

Moral status of embryo

Commentators on the moral status of the embryo have viewed the embryo anywhere from being human and worthy of respect as a person[10,12] to being human matter only, which is not alive in any personal sense.[24,25] Kass maintains that embryos clearly are biologically alive, even at the blastocyst stage. He points out that "nascent" lives are deliberately created with the knowledge that they will be intentionally destroyed or discarded. Kass emphasizes that "the human embryo is not humanly nothing. It is, at least, potential humanity ... and not to be treated as mere stuff or as mere meat."[12(p4)] Therefore he does not support unregulated laboratory in vitro fertilization research.

Fletcher's willingness to approve laboratory research with human embryos is based on his belief that the desired end justifies the means in this particular case. He further asserts that the early human embryo is not a person because it is precerebral and incapable of higher brain function because it does not possess self-awareness, memory, a sense of time or futurity, or a capacity for love or interpersonal relationship.[24,25] On the basis of this mode of reasoning, it would not be immoral to procreate human embryos in the laboratory for the sole purposes of laboratory research, after which they would be destroyed.

Informed consent of donors

The ethical question of informed consent of the sperm and egg donors has been a key concern for some ethicists.[6,10,11]

It is not clear whether persons who have allowed their gametes to be used in this research truly gave informed consent or whether consent was even obtained. For example, some oocytes may be obtained from the ovaries of women who have had surgical removal of their ovaries for medical reasons. Should or did these women give consent for their gametes to be used in laboratory research? How did gamete donors come to volunteer? What have they been told or not told about the planned research? Have some infertile couples been coerced into donating their gametes for research because they have been made to feel obligated because of the hope that they might somehow reap the benefits of such research?

No matter how well intentioned the investigator, a person's wishes should be considered and respected when experimentation on his or her body tissues, particularly on gametes, is conducted. This also is true and applicable when clinical in vitro fertilization research is done. Women who have their ovaries removed during surgical procedures should be given the option of deciding whether their eggs can be used for laboratory research. Laboratory personnel should thoroughly inform egg or sperm donors about the specific type of research that will be conducted with the use of their gametes. The personnel should then obtain their written consent. For example, some individuals may not object to research with their gametes in which the scientist will study the physiology and maturation of the embryo to further develop knowledge about embryology and teratogenesis. However, the same individuals might object vehemently if their gametes were going to be used in cloning experiments or development of chimeras, in perfecting the technology of ectogenesis with extracorporeal gestation, or in transfers of embryos to human or animal surrogate gestational mothers. All persons should be allowed to maintain control over what is to happen to their bodies and to their gametes.

IMPLICATIONS FOR WOMEN, THE FAMILY, AND SOCIETY

This article has reviewed the potential uses of in vitro fertilization and some of the issues and questions raised about the application of the procedure. The next logical step is to turn to the implications that this technology could have for those who are likely to be most intimately affected by it: women and families. Because experimentation and clinical applications of in vitro fertilization are likely to proceed, the technique is likely to become more refined, risks for the woman and fetus are likely to decrease, and acceptance and use of the procedure are likely to become somewhat more widely spread. But what may all of this mean? What options or problems can the use of in vitro fertilization incur for those who choose it?

In vitro fertilization, with its potential for facilitating cloning, mastery of the genetic code, and development of chimeras, has the same potential for harnessing good and evil as the technology of nuclear energy. The widespread use of in vitro fertilization is likely to have a major influence on women, the family structure, and, consequently, on the social and political structure of society as a whole. In vitro fertilization can raise substantial questions relating to the status of women, family

As long as in vitro fertilization remains costly and complex, its impact is likely to be limited.

relationships, rights to child support, and rights of inheritance. However, it can be expected that as long as in vitro fertilization remains costly and complex, its impact is likely to be limited.[26]

Intramarital—and extramarital—gametes

The treatment of intramarital infertility will probably be among the most common therapeutic uses of clinical in vitro fertilization. This, of course, would involve the fertilization of the wife's egg with sperm from her husband and a subsequent embryo transfer to the wife for gestation. This seems reasonable as long as the risks are not great for the woman and fetus involved. But who is to say that the procedure will or should be limited to the use of intramarital gametes?

There is no reason why the embryo must be transferred to the uterus of the same woman from whom the egg was originally obtained. A surrogate gestational mother may be employed to carry the biological mother's fetus to term and deliver it. This could be a possible option for women who have functioning ovaries but whose uterine environment is not sufficient for the implantation and gestation of a child, or for women who have had a hysterectomy but have intact ovaries. Egg donors could supply oocytes for fertilization by the husband's sperm for those women who for some reason could not supply oocytes for fertilization themselves but could carry the child to term in their own uterus after "prenatal embryo adoption." Clinical use of in vitro fertilization will probably rely on donor oocytes that have been frozen and stored in a manner analogous to the storage of sperm from donor insemination. It can be expected that egg and embryo banks will be established in the future, similar to already existing sperm banks. This could reduce the necessity for repeated operations on the same woman to obtain oocytes.

This approach to treating infertility raises legal and social questions for women and their mates. The number of women who are infertile for reasons other than blocked oviducts make it extremely likely that in vitro fertilization will not be confined to intramarital cases. A study of college undergraduates indicates that some persons would not be adverse to using donor oocytes to treat infertility.[27] Undoubtedly some couples will find the potential for prenatal adoption and the use of surrogate gestational mothers quite appealing. There is some concern that this could lead to new business ventures that could exploit women in the process of remedying some couples' infertility and that some single women, widows, and lesbians might choose this option for becoming parents. In addition, women such as actresses who do not want to burden themselves with a pregnancy, interrupt their career, or distend their figure with a pregnancy could hire a surrogate gestational mother to endure the pregnancy for them for a fee. What social implication could this have for women? Surely there are "enough poor women available to form a caste of childbearers" and egg donors for pay.[10(p36)]

What legal implications would such practices as prenatal embryo adoption and surrogate gestational motherhood have for all of those concerned? Who would be the legal parents? What would be the legal rights of the egg donor, the surrogate mother, or the child? With the high rate of divorce today, the practice of prenatal embryo adoption could present a complex dilemma for a couple who might choose to discontinue a marriage at some later time. There are presently no answers for these questions, particularly because the legal ramifications of artificial insemination by a donor are still vague after some 40 years in which the procedure has been in practice.

Psychological consequences for donor or surrogate mother

There is little doubt that prenatal embryo adoption and surrogate gestational motherhood can be respectfully and humanely practiced. But what are the psychological consequences for the woman who chooses to donate an egg or who serves as a surrogate gestational mother? Will her psychological burden be greater than the benefits garnered from participation in this practice? Could relatives be pressured to donate eggs or serve as surrogate gestational mothers without truly desiring such roles? What if the egg donor or womb-lending surrogate mother desires to keep the child once it is born? The questions are numerous and complex. Conflict, guilt, and confusion are likely to result. The legal rights and responsibilities of the egg donor, surrogate gestational mother, and the recipient parents will have to be clarified and defined. There also is a need for more research to increase understanding of the meaning of motherhood, womanhood, sexuality, and childbearing so that society can better understand—and deal with—the ramifications of the various practices of in vitro fertilization.

Family relations and government policy

In vitro fertilization and the potential for eugenic controls that it could make possible may have a deep impact on family structure and family relationships. It is doubtful that this technology will create a society of free-floating persons, grown in vitro without family attachments or responsibilities. The family may have a different kind of relationship to the state, and there could be a marked modification in the decision-making and planning processes of the government. It is not likely that society can simultaneously maintain individual freedom and an effective eugenic program. Therefore the potential for government-controlled eugenic control boards seems small, but one may reasonably assume that the government may possibly limit the nature of laboratory in vitro fertilization research and clinical applications as it has in the past.

In the final analysis each person's morals and values will help dictate the extent to which that individual will be willing to become involved in clinical in vitro fertilization procedures or to allow his or her gametes to be used in laboratory in vitro fertilization research. The choices and responses to in vitro fertilization can be expected to vary widely. All individuals who become involved in such practices—

The government may possibly limit the nature of laboratory in vitro fertilization.

the recipient parents, sperm and egg donors, surrogate gestational mothers, and nurses and other health care providers giving assistance—must be aware of how such practices fit into their own morals and values and understand the extent to which they are willing to participate. At the same time nurses and other health care providers should be accepting of those who have decided to participate in various clinical and laboratory in vitro fertilization procedures regardless of their personal feelings.

CONCLUSION

In vitro fertilization opens several options of which nurses should be aware. As this technology becomes perfected and increases in its acceptance and use, nurses are likely to become intimately involved in the care of persons who may be weighing whether they should become involved with the procedure as recipients of a therapeutic option for infertility or as egg donors for laboratory research. These options may be accepted as blessings by some persons, but they also may be threatening for others. In vitro fertilization raises as many questions as it seemingly provides answers and solutions for. Nurses need to be aware of the possible opportunities and dilemmas raised by this technologic advancement.

REFERENCES

1. Steptoe PC, Edwards RG: Reimplantation of a human embryo with subsequent tubal pregnancy. *Lancet* 1:880-882, 1976.
2. Edwards RG, Bavister BD, Steptoe PC: Early stages of fertilization in vitro of human oocytes matured in vitro. *Nature* 221:632-635, 1969.
3. Edwards RG, Steptoe PC, Purdy JM: Fertilization and cleavage in vitro of preovulator human oocytes. *Nature* 227:1307-1309, 1970.
4. Steptoe PC, Edwards RG, Purdy JM: Human blastocysts grown in culture. *Nature* 229:132-133, 1971.
5. Steptoe PC, Edwards RG: Laparoscopic recovery of preovulatory human oocytes after priming of ovaries with gonadotrophins. *Lancet* 1:683-689, 1970.
6. Kass LR: Babies by means of in vitro fertilization: Unethical experiments on the unborn? *N Engl J Med* 285:1174-1179, 1971.
7. Arrata WS: *Textbook of Gynecology.* Philadelphia: Lea Febiger, 1977.
8. Edwards RG, Sharpe DJ: Social values and research in human embryology. *Nature* 231:87-91, 1971.
9. National Research Council, Assembly of Behavioral and Social Sciences, Committee on the Life Sciences and Social Policy. *Assessing Biomedical Technologies: An Inquiry into the Nature of the Process.* Washington, DC, National Academy of Sciences, 1975.
10. Kass LR: Making babies—The new biology and the "Old" morality. *Public Interest* 26:18-56, 1972.
11. Ramsey P: Shall we "reproduce"? II. Rejoinders and future forecast. *JAMA* 220:1480-1485, 1972.
12. *A Conversation with Dr. Leon Kass: The Ethical Dimensions of In Vitro Fertilization.* Washington, DC, American Enterprise Institute for Public Policy Research, 1979.
13. Kass LR: Making babies revisited. *Public Interest* 54:32-60, 1979.
14. Hellegars AE, McCormick RA: Unanswered questions on test tube life. *America* 139:74-78, August 1978.
15. Ramsey P: Shall we "reproduce"? I. The medical ethics of in vitro fertilization. *JAMA* 220:1346-1350, 1972.
16. Huxley A: *Brave New World.* New York, Harper & Row, 1946.
17. Lappé M: Ethics at the center of life: Protecting vulnerable subjects. *Hastings Cen Rep* 8:11-13, October 1978.
18. Robertson JA: In vitro conception and harm to the unborn. *Hastings Cen Rep* 8:13-14, October 1978.
19. Toulmin S: In vitro fertilization: Answering the ethical objections. *Hastings Cen Rep* 8:9-11, October 1978.
20. Edwards RG: Fertilization of human eggs in vitro: Morals, ethics and the law. *Q Rev Biol* 49:3-26, 1974.
21. Etzioni A: Sex control, science, and society. *Science* 161:1107-1112, 1968.
22. Jones A, Bodmer WF: *Our Future Inheritance: Choice or Chance?* London, Oxford University Press, 1974.
23. Davis BD: Prospects for genetic intervention in man. *Science* 170:1279-1283, 1970.
24. Fletcher J: New beginnings in life: A theologian's response, in Hamilton MP (ed): *The New Genetics and the Future of Man.* Grand Rapids, Mich, William B. Eerdmans Publishing Co, 1972, pp 78-89.
25. Fletcher J: Ethical aspects of genetic controls: Designed genetic changes in man, in Kittrie N et al. (eds): *Medicine, Law and Public Policy.* New York, AMS Press, Inc, 1975, Vol 1, pp 569-581.
26. Grad FP: New beginnings in life: A lawyer's response, in Hamilton, MP (ed): *The New Genetics and the Future of Man.* Grand Rapids, Mich, William B. Eerdmans Publishing Co, 1972, pp 64-77.
27. Matteson RL, Terranova G: Social acceptance of new techniques of child conception. *J Soc Psychol* 101:225-229, 1977.

Resolving Interpersonal Value Conflicts

Milton Meux, Ph.D.
Bureau of Educational Research
University of Utah
Salt Lake City, Utah

VALUE CONFLICT pervades many aspects of social life at every level of the social unit—individual, group, community and society. With the recent changes in our society, however, these value conflicts seem to have increased in intensity, complexity and importance. Thus value conflict, which (as all conflict) has always been a stressor, has now become even more of a stressor. That conflict is a stressor, of course, needs no scientific documentation, since at one time or another we have all experienced the feelings of frustration, confusion, hostility, bitterness, resentment, estrangement, impotence and lowered self-confidence and self-esteem that accompany conflict.

The author gratefully acknowledges the assistance on this conceptualization over the past few years by his colleagues Terry Applegate, Jerry Coombs, Keith Evans, Mike Parsons, Bob Tucker and Bill Whisner. The author would also like to thank Gabe Della Piana, George Endo, Keith Evans and Bill Whisner for their helpful suggestions in writing this article. None of them, of course, are responsible for the deficiencies remaining in the conceptualization and its formulation here.

Although a variety of conceptualizations and practical approaches have been developed for the resolution of value conflicts, none seems to meet a wide range of both theoretical and practical criteria (e.g., theoretical criteria for the soundness of the concepts of value and value conflict in the underlying theory of value, and practical criteria for materials and strategies concerning whether they are usable for real value conflicts, ethical, general, individualized and inexpensive).

This article presents a conceptualization for the resolution of interpersonal value conflicts that meets a variety of these theoretical and practical criteria. This conceptualization emphasizes the role of rational self-legislation by participants in a value conflict in choosing a course of action to resolve the value conflict that will realize the highest value chosen by the participants. (For convenience, we present only two participants in a value conflict.)

This self-legislation conceptualization is most useful when participants in a value conflict want to effect a resolution of the value conflict that is of the highest value to them individually or jointly. In these cases the conceptualization provides ways for the participants to conceive the situation and to carry out their aim. Participants do not or should not always have such an aim, but at times they will. In long-term relations (e.g., the family) or stable health care systems it may be important for a variety of reasons to achieve a situation that realizes the highest value. This may include the participants viewing the value conflict situation as an important occasion to engage in rational self-legislation to further their self-development as persons.

In trying to improve the theoretical adequacy of this conceptualization, it has become increasingly clear that the fundamental relations between the self and a person's values and valuing processes must be considered. That such relations exist is made clear from everyday experience and from a number of value theories such as that of Werkmeister[1]—a self-legislation or self-realization theory and thus a holistic theory—and of Parker.[2] In both of these value theories the self has a central role. In fact the conceptualization presented here can be viewed as an extension of Werkmeister's value theory to the resolution of interpersonal value conflict.

CHARACTERISTICS OF SELF

Before clarifying the nature of rational self-legislation, it will be helpful to briefly describe the characteristics of self in this conceptualization. The reflexive nature of the self is perhaps its most fundamental characteristic, and probably the only one agreed upon by almost all self theorists. The self is both experiencer and experienced, both the I and the me, both $subject$ and $object$. This reflexiveness is, in Werkmeister's terms, the "inner duality of self-reflective experience which characterizes the whole of human existence."[1(p16)] Diggory's notation helps to express this reflexiveness: $X \ldots o \ldots X$. The first X is an agent, the self as subject; the o is some operation; and the second X is the object of the operation or the self as object.[3(p65)]

The characteristics of self as subject, the type of operations, and the characteristics of self as object allowed in the concept are what distinguish one concept of self from another. The concept of self presented here is rather broad, but agrees with ordinary use of the concept, with Werkmeister[1] and with some self theorists. Self as subject includes the immediate experience of self both as agent and as the experiencer (Smith's acting and experiencing I[4(p1058)]). Operations include single operations, such as reflective abstracting, comparing, redirecting, balancing, and integrating, and sets of these operations. Examples of sets of operations, which are like "roles," are diagnosing, observing, judging, adjudicating and legislating.

Self as object includes the products of reflective abstraction from the self-as-subject's experience (the "contents" of experience) such as perceptions, cognitions, beliefs, meanings, values, drives, felt needs, preferences, attitudes and feelings.

Thus in this broad concept, self as subject can engage in a variety of operations on self as object, ranging from passive to active operations, and from isolated elements of experience to broad systems (e.g., the value system). Self as subject can abstract, compare, balance, oppose, redirect, organize, integrate and in various ways exert central control over self as object (i.e., over perceptions, cognitions, desires, attitudes, feelings, values and behavior). Such a broad concept of self is needed for the variety of activities involved in rational self-legislation by the participants.

Self-legislation by a participant involves the participant placing value on some course of action and committing himself or herself to carrying out this course of action because he or she placed the value on the course of action. Therefore rational self-legislation by a participant involves the participant's placing value on a course of action on the basis of his or her rational evaluation of that course of action, and committing himself or herself to carrying out this course of action because he or she placed the value (rationally) on the course of action.

In this article rational evaluation will be regarded as essentially the same as rational value analysis (i.e., a value analysis in which the value judgment meets the following four standards of rationality stated and defended in Coombs)[5(p18)]:

1. The purported facts supporting the judgment must be true or well confirmed.

2. The facts must be genuinely relevant (i.e., they must actually have valence for the person making the judgment).

3. Other things being equal, the greater the range of relevant facts taken into account in making the judgment, the more adequate the judgment is likely to be.

4. The value principle implied by the judgment must be acceptable to the person making the judgment.

Finally, then, rational self-legislation by the participants involves the concept of interdependence. The two participants retain their individual identities but are also dependent on each other to some extent. There is individual and joint rational evaluation of alternative courses of action, with individual and joint self-legislation of (1) the criteria for choosing an action from alternatives, (2) rationally evaluating the alternative courses of action to place a value on each and (3) participants committing themselves to the action on which the highest value was placed.

Three phases of the resolution of interpersonal value conflict are presented here: (1) A *preformulation phase*, or the value conflict situation in which the participants initially find themselves; (2) a *formulation* phase in which the participants formulate important aspects of the initial value conflict situation, especially the sources of value conflict; and (3) the *resolution* phase in which the participants engage in a variety of activities selected and organized to have instrumental value for the rationally self-legislated course of action to resolve the value conflict that will realize the highest value to the participants.

Fact-assembly charts and excerpts from a transcript of an attempt at resolving a value conflict concerning gun control laws are provided to illustrate this conceptualization. Although this attempt did not completely resolve the value conflict, it does illustrate important parts of the conceptualization and indicates the capabilities of two people, Dee and John, with no special training in resolution of interpersonal value conflicts. This four-hour resolution attempt is partially simulated in the sense that each participant was strongly committed to his or her value judgment about gun control laws, but there was no real context of action requiring a resolution.

PREFORMULATION PHASE

The two participants are faced with an incompatibility of some action in a rather complex situation. Some of the main aspects of this complexity are discussed below.[6-8]

Participants

Because of the importance of interdependence in this conceptualization, the individual characteristics of each partici-

pant are distinguished from relations between the participants.

CHARACTERISTICS

Following are the characteristics for each participant that must be considered:

1. Values: rights held, feelings of obligation, duties believed to be important, intrinsic values attached to, benefits pursued, principles adhered to, standards to be met and rules to be followed (Various value perspectives and classifications of values help highlight basic conflicting values.[1,9] Nagel, for example, argues that obligations, rights, utility, perfectionistic ends and private projects are basic value types; differences among them are difficult to resolve—much more so than differences within the types.[9]);

2. Belief systems, especially beliefs about the incompatible action constituting the value conflict and other aspects of the situation;

3. Attitudes, feelings, needs, concerns, preferences, perceptions, frames of reference relevant to the incompatible action or other aspects of the situation felt or believed to be relevant;

4. Feelings of frustration, hostility and antagonism specific to the situation; and

5. Capabilities and dispositions of each participant for self-reflection, including self-awareness, self-evaluation and self-modification.

RELATIONS

Following are the relations between the participants that must be considered:

1. Prior relationships,[6] including interaction patterns[7];

2. Capabilities and dispositions for *joint* self-reflection and self-direction;

3. Capabilities and dispositions for per-spective-taking.

In the value conflict example the partici-pants, Dee and John, are concerned with gun control. Resolution of the value conflict is facilitated by a moderator, the author of this article. Dee and John were students in a graduate seminar on values with the author several weeks before participating in this resolution attempt, and so became well acquainted. Their relations were in general congenial and agreeable. They had infor-mally discussed a variety of topics, which helped identify the value conflict about gun control and some of their reasons, basic concerns about freedom, life, safety and possible actions that could be taken.

Conditions Influencing the Value Conflict

Other conditions influencing the value conflict are discussed by Deutsch,[6] includ-ing the nature of the issue, such as scope, rigidity and formulation; social environ-ment, such as facilities and restraints; and interested audiences to the value conflict, including relations to participants and each other.

In general, then, the preformulation phase is characterized by a complex mixture of contrasting factors, such as causes of and the participant's reasons for the action, participant-controlled activities and passive undergoings, objective and subjective aspects such as environment and self, implicitly and explicitly formu-lated aspects of the situation, and eliciting subjectively held values and judging the relevance of values to the situation (e.g., rights that might be violated). Clearly the reflexive self is involved in a variety of ways in such a situation.

As a result of different combinations and weightings of all the factors in the preformulation phase, the participants have placed opposing values on the incompatible action. That is, the opposing values placed on the action produce the incompatibility. Whether a participant has formulated explicitly his or her reasons for the value placed on the action, it is clear that in some sense the participants have different reasons for their valuings. For example, one participant may place nega-tive value on an action because it violates rights, whereas the other participant may place positive value on the same action because it confers many benefits on people. Or one participant may feel that an action has great value because it fulfills his or her obligations and respects the rights of all involved, whereas the other partici-pant places a negative value on the same action because it denies benefits to many people (negative utility) and interferes with the participant's own projects.

With this brief characterization of the situation confronting the participants, activities that enable the participants to begin intervening favorably in their own value conflict are now discussed.

FORMULATION PHASE

The fundamental reflexive characteristic of self—Werkmeister's inner duality of human existence[1]—enables the partici-pants to formulate the most relevant aspects of the value conflict situation so as to initiate rational self-legislation, both individually and jointly. This involves participants using their capabilities for individual and joint reflective abstraction and appraisal of the aspects of the situation, placing the aspects into perspective in a more coherent picture of the situation than the participants could have in the preformulation phase. (The participants may, of course, require or at least benefit from help by a consultant, moderator, counselor or objective third party.)

Formulation of Value Judgments

Each participant formulates his or her value judgment of the incompatible action. These opposing value judgments constitute the value conflict. Following are examples of opposing value judgments that would constitute a value conflict:

Participant A
Regular medical checkups are good
Budgeting is good
Buying a small car is desirable
Social drinking is undesirable
Telling a patient of his or her condition is wrong

Participant B
Regular medical checkups are undesirable
Budgeting is bad
Buying a small car is intolerable
Social drinking is desirable
Telling a patient of his or her condition is right

Dee and John each formulated their value judgment at the beginning of the resolution session. Dee's value judgment is that gun control is undesirable, while John's value judgment is that gun control is desirable. The difference between these opposing value judgments, then, is the value conflict. They formulate their value judgments in the following passage:

Moderator: OK, John, what's your initial value judgment?
John: I'd like to see some sort of rather strict gun control law that would reduce the number of handguns, all firearms, available to people, to citizens.
Moderator: OK. So your value judgment would be something like: Strict gun control is desirable. Something like that?
John: Yes. Strict gun control.
Moderator: Dee, what is your initial value judgment?
Dee: I do not feel that gun control is desirable.
Moderator: So your initial value judgment is: Gun control is undesirable.

Formulation of Value Analyses

Each participant is capable of formulating his or her basis, support or reasons for his or her value judgment. We call this evaluation or value reasoning a *value analysis.*

A value analysis performs a number of distinct tasks, such as clarifying the value question, gathering purported facts to support the value judgment, assessing the adequacy of the purported facts, assessing the relevance of the purported facts and testing the value principle as a whole by means of a number of tests.[10]

Since the value judgments of two participants in a value conflict are opposed, the difference must be due to differences between the participants in one or more of the above tasks in a value analysis.[10(p29)] These differences, then, must be *the direct sources* of the value conflict (see boxed material).

FACT-HIGHLIGHTING FORMULATIONS

There are various ways of formulating a value analysis. Some formulations tend to highlight the *factual* aspects of a value analysis, such as the facts a participant has included, the quality of evidence for factual claims, how the facts are ranked in importance by a participant, whether they support a negative or positive value judgment and how a single value or various values might be relevant to a single fact. An example of this kind of fact-highlighting formulation is presented in the fact-assembly charts used by Dee and John in formulating their value analyses (see Tables 1 and 2). (See Applegate and Evans for examples of such formulations in value analysis, usable in a variety of practical settings.[11])

Dee and John each completed a fact-assembly chart before the first session.[10,12] A comparison of the two charts (Tables 1 and 2) clearly depicts one of the most important sources of value conflicts— differences in the purported facts of the participants. Dee's chart presents mostly negative facts (i.e., facts supporting her negative value judgment about gun control). On the other hand, John's chart presents mostly positive facts (i.e., facts supporting his positive value judgment about gun control).

VALUE-HIGHLIGHTING FORMULATIONS

Other ways of formulating a value analysis tend to highlight the values felt, perceived or believed to be important in supporting or giving reasons for a value judgment. Such formulations would show what the values are, how a participant ranks such values in importance for this situation, and, given some value, which fact or facts are seen as relevant to that value. For example, the fact-assembly chart in Coombs and Meux shows the basic values (concerns) for a participant in evaluating the use of DDT, the facts relevant for each value and the *subsidiary*

TASKS IN PERFORMING INDIVIDUAL VALUE ANALYSIS	CORRESPONDING DIRECT SOURCES OF VALUE CONFLICT AS A DIFFERENCE IN ONE OR MORE TASKS
1. Identifying and clarifying the value question.	1. Differences in the interpretation of the value question.
2. Assembling ... purported facts.	2. Differences in the purported facts assembled.
3. Assessing the truth of purported facts.	3. Differences in the assessed truth of purported facts.
4. Clarifying the relevance of facts.	4. Differences in the relevance of facts.
5. Arriving at a tentative value judgment.	5. Differences in the tentative value judgments.
6. Testing the acceptability of the value principle implied by the value judgment and facts.	6. Differences in testing the acceptability of value principles.

TABLE 1

Fact-Assembly Chart Formulated by Dee for Gun Control Resolution
(Value Judgment: Gun Control is Undesirable)

Positive Facts	Rank	Negative Facts	Criteria for Negative Facts
1. Handguns were used in 10,323, or 53%, of the murders committed in 1973.	1	On a per capita basis the highest ownership of guns is in Switzerland. Crime rate one of lowest in world.	Every person should own and keep his/her gun and ammunition.
2. From 1964-1973, 613 policemen were killed with guns.	2	Switzerland lowest increase in crime rate in Europe.	
3. 47% of the handguns used in crimes were "Saturday Night Specials."	3	There is no proof that registration will lower crime rate.	Harrington—Program control.
4. 1.8 million handguns are manufactured in the U.S. each year; 1.3 million are "Saturday Night Specials."	4	Most restrictive laws in U.S. are in N.Y., Wash., D.C., Detroit, and Chicago—These 4 cities account for 20% of homicides.	
5. Crime is increasing all over U.S.	5	Gun that killed R. Kennedy was registered.	
	6*	2nd amendment—"A well regulated militia being necessary to the security of a free state, the right of the people to keep and bear arms shall not be infringed."	
	7*	N.Y. 1968 did a study of cost of processing one application—$72.78. Estimate today would be $100.00.	
	8	At above rate just to register handguns in U.S. each year would be $4 to $5 million.	
	9*	Highland Park, Mich. tried an educational experiment. Trained businessmen in use of guns—and advertised their use in stores. Robberies dropped from 1.5 a day to zero in four months.	
	10*	In Wash., D.C. in one year (1974) 180 brought to trial for illegal possession of gun—only 14 convicted.	
	11	In N.Y. only one in six gun crimes sentenced to jail.	
	12*	Colin Greenwood—In Study-Gun controls ineffective in dealing with serious crime. Tremendous increase armed crimes due to social factors. More willing to commit violent crimes. More illegal guns than legal guns now in England.	
	13	Little effect because handguns used in only 4% of serious crimes.	

*Five most important facts.

TABLE 2

Fact-Assembly Chart Formulated by John for Gun Control Resolution
(Value Judgment: Strict Gun Control is Desirable)

Negative Facts	Rank	Positive Facts	Criteria for Positive Facts
1. Despite stiff gun control laws in England the percentage increase of indictable offenses each year in which a gun is used is high. From 1968–1969: 31%.	1*	In 1974 there were 27,000 people killed by guns in U.S. (All deaths by guns. *Reader's Digest*, 1975.)	Instruments that result in the deaths of 27,000 citizens each year should be very tightly controlled and not readily available for use.
2. Federal Gun Control Act of 1968 banned importation of inexpensive handguns. This has not worked since parts have been imported and assembled in U.S.	2	Every 19 minutes an American is killed with a handgun.	Any instrument involved in the murder of over 10,000 Americans each year should be controlled from easy availability.
3. Approximately 55,107 work days are required to maintain and enforce the gun control law in England.	3	In 1973 there were 10,340 homicides in U.S. involving handguns.	Any instrument used in a very high percentage of murders, i.e., 67%, should not be readily available for use by anyone.
	4*	67% of all murders were committed with firearms in U.S. in 1975. (*Reader's Digest*, 1975.)	
	5	*U.S. (1963):* Rate of homicides: 2.7 per 100,000. Rate of suicides: 5.1 per 100,000. Rate of accidental deaths: 1.2 per 100,000. *England and Wales (1963):* Rate of homicides: .05 per 100,000. Rate of suicides: .34 per 100,000. Rate of accid. deaths: .16 per 100,000. England and Wales have uniform, strict gun control laws.	Any gun control law that reduces deaths by firearms is desirable. Any instrument intended for the protection of its owner that is more likely to prove harmful to the owner should be controlled.
	6*	A gun kept by a civilian for protection is 6 times more likely to kill a family member or friend than an intruder or attacker. (*Reader's Digest*, 1975.)	
	7	In Philadelphia murder by firearms reduced 9% against national average after instituting gun control law involving permit system in which fingerprinting and photo necessary for purchase. Felons not allowed to purchase firearms. Three hundred twenty-three felons denied permits in one year.	Any law that reduces murders by firearms 9% is good.
	8	With strict gun control laws the number of firearms registered in England is generally decreasing each year. A decrease of 3% was noted from 1968 to 1969.	Any law that reduces the number of firearms is beneficial.

continued.

TABLE 2 (cont'd.)

Negative Facts	Rank	Positive Facts	Criteria for Positive Facts
	9	In 1975 there were 40 million handguns in U.S. (est.)	
	10*	Two million handguns sold each year in U.S. (*Reader's Digest*, 1975.)	
	11*	Gallup and Harris polls indicate two-thirds of citizens favor more effective gun control laws, including (1) registration, (2) licensing of gun users.	Any proposal that gains majority favor of public should be strongly considered for adoption.
*Five most important facts.			

value judgment for each value (i.e., the presence or quantity of *that* kind of value judged by the participant to be characteristic of the use of DDT).[10(p43)] For this person the use of DDT is highly detrimental in ecologic value, much less useful and effective in economic value, is risky and self-defeating in practical value and probably dangerous in health value.

COMPARISON OF FACT-HIGHLIGHTING AND VALUE-HIGHLIGHTING FORMULATIONS

Both fact- and value-highlighting formulations have advantages and disadvantages. Some advantages of the fact-highlighting formulation are that (1) it seems to require less abstraction from the concrete value conflict situation and thus may be more "natural" for participants; (2) it requires only a simple judgment of whether a fact is relevant to the value analysis; (3) many value conflicts may be resolved by focusing only on the factual sources of the value conflict; and (4) specific practical procedures of this type have been developed by Applegate and Evans[11] for individual value analyses.

One advantage of the value-highlighting formulation is that it makes more explicit the values or perspectives on which basis the relevance of any fact is judged, the subsidiary value judgments that can be viewed as components of and synthesized into the value judgment.

Most important, however, is that the set of subsidiary value judgments for a participant can be viewed as a clear way of expressing the values of the participant that are *realized* in the action. Thus this is called the *value realization pattern*. The differences between the participants in their value realization patterns provide a clear way to pinpoint the *value* sources of the value conflict and to diagnose whether these differences can be sufficiently reduced on this action so as to resolve the value conflict or whether another action must be selected or constructed. Another use of the value realization pattern for each action is to facilitate a direct and easy comparison with the *value criteria pattern* formulated as an *end* by the participants (see discussion on *end*). This value criteria pattern is the basis for judging whether an action will resolve the conflict (at a minimum) and whether an action can realize other values important to the participants.

Because of the importance of value-highlighting in resolving value conflicts and to facilitate comparison of the fact-highlighting and value-highlighting formulations, the fact-assembly charts of Dee and John have been reconstructed (Figure 1).

The fact-assembly charts in Tables 1 and 2 have been simplified by using a single term to represent a value, listing only the numbers of the facts from Tables 1 and 2, combining two or three values distinguished in the transcript, and arranging the columns differently to facilitate comparison of the value sources of conflict. Almost all of the five values have a serious difference, and the values are also ranked differently by Dee and John. It is also clear that differences in the purported facts for the top-ranked values are an important source of the value conflict.

Indirect Sources of the Value Conflict

Sources of the value conflict other than differences between value analyses of participants are also important, but only insofar as they influence or are relevant to how a participant performs a value analysis. These are *indirect sources* of the value conflict, for example: (1) a participant's perceptions of the incompatible action may influence his or her beliefs about the incompatible action or the degree of incompatibility; (2) prejudice may influence a participant's feelings and attitudes about the relevance of a fact; (3) a "concrete individual" may have difficulty

understanding the perspective or role of another person[10]; and (4) stress may overload either participant in a variety of ways, especially restricting the range of relevant facts a participant can take into account, thus biasing the value judgment.

These indirect sources include many of the conditions considered necessary or sufficient to resolve conflicts, thus facilitating or inhibiting conditions in both the initial value conflict situation and in resolution attempts.[6-8]

The conditions for the formulation phase involved Dee and John formulating their value analyses out of class, including research in the library. These conditions seemed optimal, although both felt they could have used more time.

What has been accomplished in this formulation phase is that, by the participants' formulating the important aspects of the initial value conflict situation, they have transformed it—with its mixture of active and passive, objective and subjective, and self as both subject and object—to a situation that facilitates rational appraisal and deliberation,[1(p129)] an essential part of rational self-legislation.

RESOLUTION PHASE

As a result of the formulation phase the participants have formulated what they see to be the relevant aspects of the initial value conflict situation, especially the direct sources of the value conflict, the subsidiary value judgments. This formulation includes both the reflective abstraction necessary to self and the identification of aspects of the situation external to self.

FIGURE 1.   Reconstructed Fact-Assembly Charts for Value-Highlighting Formulation

Dee's Value Judgment:
Gun Control is Undesirable

Facts (−)	(+)	Value	Value Ranking	SVJ*
9	4	Freedom	1	Very threatening
	1-5	Life	3	Questionable effectiveness
1, 10, 12 5, 11, 13		Legal	2	Anti-constitutional and ineffective
	3, 5	Safety	5	Relatively ineffective
7, 8		Cost	4	High

John's Value Judgment:
Strict Gun Control is Desirable

SVJ*	Value	Value Ranking	Facts (+)	(−)
Only somewhat threatening	Freedom	3	10 3, 5, 8, 9	
Highly desirable	Life	1	1, 4, 6 2, 7	
Somewhat effective	Legal	4	11	First fact Second fact
—†	Safety	2		
Somewhat high	Cost	5		Third fact

(+) = Positive
(−) = Negative
*SVJ = Subsidiary Value Judgment
†No SVJ given because no facts in fact-assembly chart for this value. However, the transcript indicated this high ranking of the safety Value.
Note: First row of facts are the five most important as shown in Tables 1 and 2.

As a whole, this formulation helps the participants achieve a balanced and coherent understanding and appraisal of the initial value conflict situation so as to help decide what activities should be undertaken in the resolution of the value conflict to realize the highest value possible through a rational self-legislation.

The general aim of the resolution phase, then, is for the participants to achieve rational self-legislation of some course of action that holds the highest value for the participants. Many activities can help achieve this general aim. How should we conceptualize these activities to be most helpful to the participants in achieving the general aim? Or how can we conceptualize the activities to maximize the instrumental value of the activities for this general aim? Following are several main considerations:

1. In order for the participants to rationally self-legislate the highest value, they need some concept of a rationally chosen end. Thus the participants need a conception of the range of choices for the end and how to rationally evaluate these in order to select and self-legislate their end.

2. In order for the participants to rationally self-legislate a means to achieve the end, and to realize the values in the end, the participants need some concept of the means possible. Thus the participants need a conception of the range of means to be considered and how to rationally evaluate these in order to self-legislate their means.

3. In order for the participants to manage conditions that will facilitate and not inhibit carrying out the central activities in the first and second considerations,

the participants need a conception of conditions relevant for these purposes.

4. Other things being equal, the more adequately the activities are carried out, singly and in combinations, the greater their instrumental value for the general aim. Thus in order for participants to do this, they need a conception of the relevant criteria of adequacy (e.g., rules, standards, principles, procedures, strategies) for these activities.

5. In order for the participants to more clearly understand their possible operations on themselves (self as subject operating on self as object) and on the value conflict situation external to self, the activities can be conceptualized as operations on some content to meet a criterion of adequacy. This should also help the participants increase their self-control over the processes or activities in the resolution phase and thereby increase their self-legislation.

What does it mean to conceptualize an activity as an operation on some content to meet a criterion of adequacy? This will be examined briefly; how this conceptualization helps meet the five considerations or requirements listed above will then be discussed.

Viewing an activity as an operation on some content to meet a criterion of adequacy is an extension of the concept of an activity as an operation on some content.[13] Thus in reformulating the problem the operation is *reformulating* and the content is *the problem*. In evaluating an end the operation is *evaluating* and the content is an *end*. In fractionating an issue the operation is *fractionating* and the content is an *issue*.

However, not only does an activity

involve an operation on a content, but it also can be evaluated in terms of its adequacy on the basis of one or more criteria, rules, standards or principles. For example, reformulating the problem can be judged on the basis of how well it incorporates the underlying conflict between the participants. Evaluating an end can be assessed on the basis of how well it meets the standards of rationality discussed earlier in this article. Fractionating an issue can be evaluated on the basis of how well it simplifies the value conflict or facilitates reaching an agreement on some subissues. *Criteria of adequacy* is used here as an umbrella term for all these rules, standards and principles; it also is used for sets or combinations of activities such as strategies, procedures, algorithms and plans.

Criteria of adequacy for operations include conjecturing, clarifying, evaluating, and modifying. When evaluating operations are rational, the first and second requirements listed above can be met. Criteria of adequacy for content includes elements of the resolution situation (especially participants, end, means and conditions) and relations between the participants. The first (end), second (means), third (conditions), and fifth (self vs external to self) requirements listed above can then be met.

Criteria of adequacy can be distinguished as single activities and sets (combinations, sequences or hierarchies) of activities. This helps meet the fourth requirement listed above.

Content, operations and criteria of adequacy of an activity are now discussed to facilitate understanding of how partici-pants achieve rational self-legislation of a means of the highest value.

Content of an Activity

Two types of content of an activity are important: (1) *elements* of the resolution situation such as the participants, problem, end, means or conditions (These elements are important because they show the locus of *possible* changes in the situation that can both remove the initial incompatibility and increase the value of the situation if modified.) and (2) *relations* between the participants such as the differences in value analysis tasks that constitute the direct sources of the value conflict. The reduction of these differences may be an important type of activity in joint rationality.

ELEMENTS OF THE RESOLUTION SITUATION

The important elements of the resolution situation are the participants, the end, the means and the conditions. The participants (and their relevant characteristics) have already been discussed in the preformulation phase.

The end. The decision about the end involves the rationally self-legislating criteria for the highest value by means of a *value criteria pattern.*

A value criteria pattern is essentially a complex criterion or standard, with each component being some value that specifies the presence or quantity [Note: Quantity is indicated by qualifiers in the value judgment, for example, "slightly," "somewhat," and "highly."] of a value that is to be realized by any action (means) that is to resolve the value conflict. Following is an example of a value criteria pattern for an end concerning the gun control content:

- Clearly effective;
- Inexpensive;
- Not freedom-infringing;
- Safe; and
- Moral.

In order to decide on a value criteria pattern, the participants need some way of identifying the relevant values they want realized by the action they choose to resolve the value conflict. That is, it would help if the participants had some way of ensuring, or at least making plausible, that they have a wide range of relevant values in their value criteria pattern.

Although no method to ensure this is known, participants may consider for inclusion in their value criteria pattern the following value perspectives and types of values:

- Werkmeister's scale of values, increasing in extent of involvement of self: sensory pleasure, gratification of appetites, sense of well-being, satisfaction, communal living, peace of mind, joys of enterprise and creation, and sense of fulfillment (happiness)[1(pp114-117)];
- Applegate and Evans's set of ten values (concerns) found useful in their practical work in value analysis: aesthetic, ecologic, economic, effectiveness, health and safety, legal, moral/ethical, political, social and survival[11(p50)];
- Nagel's five basic types of value: obligations, rights, utility, perfectionistic ends and private commitments[9(pp129-131)];
- Nagel's list of factors to consider: economic, political, and personal liberty; equality; equity; privacy; procedural fairness; intellectual and aesthetic development; community; general utility; desert; avoidance of arbitrariness; acceptance of risk; the interests of future generations; the weight to be given to interests of other states or countries[9(p141)]; and
- Some comprehensive set of interpersonal values to include cooperation, mutual trust and understanding, fulfilling joint responsibilities, sharing, intellectual stimulation, friendship, belonging and self-transcendence.[2(p165)]

See also Edel's concept of a personal base,[14(p329)] Rescher's and Taylor's principles for classifying values,[15,16] and Oliver and Shaver's table of oft-conflicting values.[17(p142)]

For the participants' purposes, it may be helpful at times to distinguish between process and product ends and between particular and general ends.

Process-product ends. The end may involve achieving some kind of process of resolution (that is, some set of activities such as meeting the standards of rationality,[5,11,18] having equality of participation, moral/ethical activities, and self-legislation). On the other hand, the end may concern the final product of the resolution attempt: the state of affairs to be realized that meets the value criteria pattern, such as new beliefs of a participant or a modified environment. Important values in the product aspect of the value criteria pattern include effectiveness, moral/ethical values, and various benefits. It is important here for participants to distinguish individual values for each participant to realize in the resolution action from interpersonal values.

Particular-general ends. A particular end, which would include Coombs' particular objective,[18] involves resolving only the particular value conflict in the situation, that is, removing the incompatible value judgments so that action can proceed. A general end, on the other hand, goes beyond resolving the value conflict of the particular situation and may include developing one's strategies for coping with value conflicts (e.g., developing capabilities for rational value analysis),[5,10,11] modifying a participant's belief system to be more adequate or changing the environment so as to be more beneficial. All of these are intended to increase the value of the future of the system, including greater health of the participants, and thereby to at least reduce the probability of future value conflicts between the participants.

In the gun control example the most important process end is to carry out the essential aspects of a strategy much like the guaranteed minimal yearly income strategy used earlier[12] but supplemented with a search for alternative means to the incompatible action in the initial value conflict. The strategy is formulated so that it helps participants increase the rationality of their individual value judgments.

There are two kinds of product ends: *particular* and *general.* The particular end here was to resolve the initial value conflict about gun control (that John regards it as desirable and Dee as undesirable) and included clarifying the values to be sought by each participant in the resolution. The general end here was to clarify the changes needed in the relevant system, to come to some understanding of the factors involved in the problem, and for the participants to understand both their own and each other's viewpoint.

The following two passages illustrate this kind of activity—clarifying the values to be met in the end.

John: Well, I guess moral would be my primary point of view, in the sense that innocent people are being killed with firearms. That would be my primary point of view. There may be other ones involved but I haven't really considered them yet.

Moderator: OK, Dee.

Dee: I would say moral first, but economic is very important.

Moderator: OK, so you have two primary points of view with moral first. OK, is there anything else that either of you could think of that would help you clarify the value question?

John: Yes, I'd like to add that safety is also another variable here, besides moral also safety. I'm not sure if you could use that as another variable, but it seems different.

Dee: In other words, you really are not considering gun control laws as they are now? You want to come up with something that would be effective in lowering accidents and homicides during crime.

John: Right. It could be a present law that's being considered, or something else. Whatever would work and wouldn't take away too much of the freedom of individuals and be too expensive. Let me add that I mean I don't want something that's going to cost everybody $10,000 every year or something, but I'm sure we could find some solution that wouldn't have a price tag like that on it

The means. Of the possible courses of action in the value conflict situation, there may be few or many means for achieving the end. Whatever the case, the participants choose the means on the basis of how well it achieves the end; that is, how well the value realization pattern of the means meets the value criteria pattern.

Rational value realization pattern. As already indicated, the value-highlighting formulation of a value analysis produces a set of subsidiary value judgments called the value realization pattern. (Note that the *kinds* of values in the value realization pattern are the same as those in the value criteria pattern.) A *rational* value realization pattern, then, is the set of subsidiary value judgments resulting from a *rational* value analysis; that is, one that meets the standards of rationality.[5]

It is assumed that the rational value realization pattern is used as the basis for comparison with the value criteria pattern. Why? Recall that the general aim for the resolution phase involves rational evaluation. However, the less rational the value analysis, the more likely participants are to change their value judgments if they were to do a more rational value analysis. Such a value analysis will be called here a "less-than-rational" value analysis. The importance of this distinction is that the value judgment from a rational analysis may or may not be different from the value judgment from a less-than-rational value analysis. In some cases the rational and less-than-rational value analyses will have the same result; that is, the value judgments of the two participants are not incompatible. In these cases the participants are fortunate, since their decisions about whether there will be a value conflict on the action chosen to resolve the value conflict will not be in error. On the other hand, if the value judgments from the less-than-rational analyses are different from the rational value judgments, then the participants will act on their judgments erroneously. They may (1) decide that there is no more value conflict—when there really is—and carry out that action, with the cost of moving to another action or continuing with the costs already incurred with the initial action if they remain with it; or (2) decide that there is a value conflict—when there actually is not—and waste time continuing to search for an action on which there is no conflict.

There are obviously many possibilities. Deciding among all these possibilities requires some criterion of adequacy for combinations of activities, such as a strategy; this will be discussed in the section on criteria of adequacy.

Existing means vs new means. Two further distinctions are helpful to the participants. The means may exist at the onset of the value conflict or they may be new, constructed for the purposes of resolving the value conflict, as in the case of many compromises. The construction of new means may be especially important if all existing means are inadequate for resolving the value conflict, as in the case with our gun control example. Although this construction occurs frequently in everyday life, it is not considered here as a matter of course.

In the gun control example a rather large set of existing means, all of which have deficient value realization patterns because she judges them to be ineffective, is referred to by Dee; this set is more or less the focus of the initial value conflict in the first part of the resolution phase.

Dee: Either accidental or criminal. I think there are some things that can be done that I would buy into that would be parts of gun control, but not gun control as it's in the 128 laws Congress is considering now. Or the 1968 one that was passed. I think they're ineffective.

After exploring these for some time (i.e., appraising their value realization patterns), the participants found it especially helpful to construct new means of their own to meet the underlying problem and move toward resolving the value conflict. This started toward the end of the resolution phase and included examining such means as eliminating "Saturday Night Specials" and requiring education in handling guns. (This is an example of fractionating means.[19]) The following passages illustrate creating or constructing new means.

Moderator: Looking at the rest of the facts that we starred, they indicate that there is a problem here with all these guns being implicated in accidental and other deaths, that's what John's facts pretty much point to. We're going to get into the same kind of bind that other people do, that existing facts or existing gun control laws if we move to a new resolution, a new gun control law then we won't have any facts directly on the new gun control law. So we will have . . .

Dee: Maybe we could. For instance, his facts certainly indicate that "Saturday Night Specials" are used in a big percentage of street crimes and things of that sort. If we could control, outlaw, get rid of them in this country, "Saturday Night Specials," we would eliminate the kids and the people who buy a cheap gun and don't know anything about it at least, and that would be reasonable to me.

Mediator: Yeah, that's what I was going to say. Looks like that would be reasonable to assume even though there aren't any direct, hard facts on that.

John: I'd agree with that. Yeah. . . . Is it possible to have a course then when you buy a gun? You have to go through an educational program in order to purchase it—maybe pass a test and be able to demonstrate using your gun.

Mediator: I like that.

John: Demonstrate using a gun safely. I'd really like that. I think that could really be useful.

Mediator: I bet that would cut down on these accidents.

Dee: That's my idea of what education is. Yes. You have to pass the course, refreshers are fine, and everybody in the family; 'cause everybody is exposed to it. And you don't just sell a gun to somebody who doesn't have it.

Means for particular ends vs means for general ends. The means may contain activities only to achieve a particular end or may include activities for achieving a general end, which might include changing a participant's values, capabilities for a rational value analysis[11] or changing some part of the environment.

Conditions. The conditions for the resolution phase are essentially the same as the indirect sources of value conflict from the formulation phase. In the resolution phase they influence value analyses that formulate the value realization patterns just as they influenced the direct sources of value conflict. As already indicated, these conditions have been discussed considerably in the conflict resolution literature (e.g., see Deutsch's discussion of the course of destructive conflict and the course of constructive conflict).[6]

In the gun control example were a number of ground rules such as each participant completing the fact-assembly chart, using more than one session, using a moderator who would be active in attempting to minimize stress and reduce the amount of tangential discussion while allowing full relevant participation from each participant. It also included taping the discussion, which made a difference, as indicated by Dee and John in off-taping comments.

RELATIONS BETWEEN PARTICIPANTS

The second main type of content is some kind of relation between the participants such as a similarity, a difference of some kind, an authority relation or a power relation.

The sources of the value conflict—the differences in the tasks in a value analysis or the subsidiary value judgments—are one of the central relations between participants. Others would be differences in the value criteria pattern judged to be best by each participant, differences in how to construct new means and agreements on how to handle stress in the resolution phase.

The whole range of interpersonal values indicated above involve relations between the participants, including mutual trust, cooperation, friendship, mutual satisfaction in resolving the conflict and equality of participation.

In the gun control example, differences between the fact-assembly charts (e.g., in facts and in subsidiary value judgment) are examples of relations between the participants.

The concept of joint rationality essentially involves relations between the participants, both in facts agreed on, values agreed on in the value criteria pattern and the interpersonal values realized in any action, as expressed in the value realization pattern.

Operations in an Activity

There are at least four distinct kinds of operations involved in the resolution of value conflicts: conjecturing, clarifying, evaluating and modifying. The first three correspond to major types discussed earlier.[13]

CONJECTURING

Conjecturing puts forth something for consideration, to consider as a possible solution for something, as in conjecturing an interpretation of a problem, conjecturing a new means and conjecturing a new definition for a term. Examples of conjecturing are stating, producing, constructing, countering, proposing, introducing and supposing. Thus the conjecturing operations propose alternatives for consideration in reflective abstraction and are necessary for any kind of change to take place.

CLARIFYING

Clarifying operations clarify conjectures in various ways, depending on what is conjectured, so that the participants have a clearer idea of what they are confronted with that already exists in the value conflict situation or what has been conjectured for a change. Examples of clarifying are identifying, defining, inferring, describing, specifying, interpreting, perspective-taking, conceptualizing and explaining. Clarifying is an essential part of reflective abstraction, and helps participants determine what they are legislating and to what they are committing themselves.

EVALUATING

Evaluating rates, assigns or ascribes value to something, places value on things, or supports, justifies or gives reasons for ratings, value judgments and value decisions. Examples of evaluating are rating, assigning value to, challenging, appraising, assessing, deliberating, and, of course, the complex set of operations in a rational value analysis. Evaluating is clearly necessary for the participants to determine the extent to which any action realizes the participant's values (the rational value realization pattern) and to decide on a value criteria pattern, that is, all the distinct aspects of what is involved in the participants' rationally self-legislating the means with the highest value.

MODIFYING

Closely related to conjecturing are various operations that actually modify something in the situation, that is, some content. Examples of modifying are reducing, transforming, fractionating, differentiating, integrating, synthesizing, narrowing, reranking, reinterpreting and reformulating. Without the modifying operations the value conflict situation could not be changed in whatever direction the participants decide is of the highest value. Thus there could be no meaningful self-legislation.

Activities Involving Operations on Relational Content

As indicated above, one type of content is relations between the participants. Thus one way of classifying activities is on the basis of relational content.

Since one central kind of relation is the sources of value conflict, one important activity involves operations on these sources of value conflict. In the conceptualization of the resolution of value conflict,[12] resolution was essentially defined as the identification and reduction of these sources of value conflict on the initial action. Although resolution is no longer defined this way, identifying and reducing the differences in the value analysis of the two participants are still important activities in a rational self-legislation conceptualization of the resolution of value conflict. This is because, while carrying out these activities, the participants can increase both their individual and joint rationality. These activities are also important in determining whether commitment to an action should be maintained.

Carrying out the six tasks for explicitly and extensively identifying and reducing differences in the sources of their initial value conflict was the first part of the strategy used in the gun control example, especially identifying and reducing of differences in the assessed truth and relevance of the factual claims in the fact-assembly charts. The charts clearly indicate some of the sources, with the differences between Dee and John in positive and negative facts. The focus on their differences occupied 24 pages of transcript in the first part of the resolution attempt. Following are examples of three kinds of reducing differences.

1. Reducing differences in interpretation of the value question:

Moderator: OK. We're going to go through the six tasks, and the first task was going to be the clarification of the value question. John, what do you mean by your value object, strict gun control?

John: I would include all firearms—in terms of the value object, you mean, not just handguns, but since a lot of innocent people are killed with rifles and other kinds of firearms each year. So, to start, anyway, I'd say all firearms.

Moderator: OK. That's good. Dee, what would you say if you were to specify your value object?

Dee: I would have to say that, other than "Saturday Night Specials," I don't feel gun control would be of any value.

Moderator: Then your value object is gun control, other than "Saturday Night Specials." OK.

2. Reducing differences in the purported facts assembled:

Dee: I could add to that and it would help your side. I think we could in that fact go on and say that 40% of the violent crimes do use handguns. Four percent of serious crimes with guns and 40% of violent crimes—and I think that's pertinent. That should go in if we're going to be fair.

3. Reducing differences in the assessed truth of purported facts:

John: I'd really like to know where you got fact 7, too.

Dee: I got that from a [names a politician] article in *Reader's Digest* . . .

John: Well, I'm not sure if I could buy all that [names same politician as above] says; he's got a lot at stake in this thing, I guess, he may say some things that may not be completely true.

Dee: What do you disagree with, the estimate today or the study estimate that it costs $72.78 to process one application to either grant or turn down a gun registration?

John: I'm just not sure he's telling the truth, that's all.

Dee: Well, I assume we could find out if there was a study done.

John: Yeah, that's true. This is from a study, and if he didn't hire these people to do the study, and ask them to kind of help him out with some of this, finding some data on his side, I could accept it a little better, a little more.

Dee: New York City did the study. It was a study there, for their cost.

Moderator: You're concerned, John, that maybe [names same politician as above] didn't quote the study right?

John: Yeah, I guess, and propaganda. That he may be using this data . . . or he may not have quoted the study right, I guess that's what I'm worried about. I mean he is a politician. I'll accept fact 7 now. It seems reasonable and I was just kind of being picky there maybe.

Criteria of Adequacy

As indicated above, a variety of criteria of adequacy are relevant for evaluating, guiding and organizing the activities in the resolution phase (e.g., rules, standards, principles, strategies, procedures, algorithms and plans). These more or less explicit criteria are scattered throughout both the philosophical[2] and psychological literature[12,20] relevant to conflict resolution.

One important way to classify the criteria is on the basis of whether they apply to single activities relevant to some operation or element of the situation or whether they apply to sets of activities (e.g., for the entire resolution session, for only the formulation phase or only the resolution phase).

SINGLE ACTIVITIES

We have already given examples of criteria of adequacy for single activities, such as the criterion of incorporating more of the underlying conflict between the participants for evaluating the activity of reformulating a problem. Another criterion of adequacy for fractionating a means is how well it simplifies the value conflict or facilitates reaching agreement on some subissues.

OPERATIONS OR CONTENT

Relevance to operations. Criteria of adequacy may be used to evaluate conjecturing, clarifying, evaluating or modifying. For clarifying, criteria for sound conceptual analysis might be relevant, such as clarity, accord with common usage, significance, rigor and fruitfulness. For evaluating, the standards of rationality[5] are applicable anywhere in either the formulation or resolution phases and are especially important in our rational self-legislation conceptualization.

Relevance to content. Criteria of adequacy may be classified by relevance to the participants, end, means or conditions. For participants there are criteria of adequacy for evaluating the participants' beliefs when expressed as factual claims (standard of rationality no. 1 in Coombs[5] and no. 2 in Applegate and Evans[11]). There are even criteria for evaluating a participant's values, that is, criteria of "axiological adequacy"[21,22] such as clarity, consistency, generality, congruence with known fact or experience, harmony and coherence. For ends Edel suggests such criteria as attractiveness, purity, permanence, constructiveness and depth.[23(p78)] (See also his

extended discussion of the evaluation of ends.[24]) For means, many values are relevant, as discussed earlier. For conditions, Frost and Wilmot,[20] Deutsch[6] and Nye[7] summarize much of the relevant literature such as avoiding stress, reducing misconceptions and using a moderator.

Criteria of adequacy for sets of activities. Criteria of adequacy for sets of activities guide and organize an entire set of activities in all phases of the resolution of value conflict. Examples of such general criteria of adequacy are strategies, procedures, algorithms and plans. Examples of such general criteria of adequacy are Meux et al.'s strategy on guaranteed minimal yearly income and the ten-step procedure for legalization of abortion.[12]

The strategy used in the gun control example involved mainly the use of the fact-assembly charts and focusing on the first three of the six sources of value conflict specified in terms of the tasks in a value analysis discussed earlier. There was also an explicit search for means other than the initial means that produced the value conflict. This strategy is similar to the strategy used for the resolution on guaranteed minimal yearly income in Meux et al.[12] The main advantages are helping participants clarify their own and each other's position and values and helping avoid the risk of wrongly rejecting the initial incompatible action if there is a strong commitment to it.

The importance of strategies is now discussed and a seven-step procedure is presented that is based on a value-highlighting formulation of the value conflict situation.

Strategies. As discussed earlier, there are

three kinds of action possible in a situation: those having disvalue for both participants, those on which there will be a value conflict, and those judged positively by both participants, thus constituting resolution actions.

This classification is important to remember when participants try to find the best means, since participants cannot determine the type of action without a rational value analysis. To find the best means, both participants must conjecture all possible actions and perform individual and joint rational value analyses on each means in order to determine which type of action it is. This clearly presents a dilemma to the participants, since in many situations with a large number of actions there will be insufficient time or inclination to undertake both functions.

For any given action, the less rational the value analyses, the more risks the participants take in either accepting or rejecting it as a resolution action. If the participants reject an action that is actually a resolution action, they must continue to search for a resolution action, thus wasting time and ignoring a resolution action that might have provided a unique value in addition to those specified in the value criteria pattern. On the other hand, if the participants agree on a resolution action when it is actually a value conflict (or even a disvalue) action, then the participants will continue to have a value conflict with its various consequences.

Many strategies have been considered both in everyday life and in the conflict resolution literature.

One type is a *minimax* strategy that minimizes the worst risks. If the participants can determine the worst risks for their situation, they then can determine what to do. If the worst risk is to lose time and commitment in an action (e.g., the initial action or newly constructed ones), then the participants must put in extra effort on value analyses of actions so that they do not reject any mistakenly. On the other hand, if the worst mistake is to agree on a new action that then turns out to be a value conflict action (e.g., if the participants detest resolving value conflicts), then they should put in extra effort on value analyses so they do not agree mistakenly.

Another type of strategy is a *bandwith-fidelity* strategy. In the first or bandwith stage a small amount of not very reliable or valid information is obtained on a wide range of actions in order to select a few actions for further consideration; in the second or fidelity stage the selected actions are then evaluated more carefully before a final decision is made on the best action. As presented here, this strategy would amount to performing a far less than rational value analysis in the first stage on a wide range of possible actions to select a few for further consideration. In the second stage, participants would perform rational value analyses on the actions selected before deciding on the best resolution action. That is, on the actions selected, participants would determine the rational value realization pattern for each action and compare these patterns to the value criteria pattern to determine the best resolution action.

A number of helpful activities could be undertaken in the bandwith stage. For example, participants could check their two top-ranked values to determine if either has a value conflict between the participants' subsidiary value judgments. If they do, participants could identify and reduce differences in factual claims and adequacy of evidence. Then if these subsidiary value conflicts cannot be eliminated, the actions can be rejected. For example, Dee eliminated all 128 means because they are ineffective. On the other hand, if the differences can be reduced even further with more activities that help reduce differences, then the action should be included for further consideration in the fidelity stage. Activities for identifying and reducing differences, which were the central part of Meux et al.'s earlier conceptualization,[12] seem most useful in the bandwith stage of a strategy. This is essentially what happened in the gun control example. These activities also seem useful in clarifying the other participant's position, understanding the other person and identifying to some degree what might be important values in each participant's value criteria pattern and in their joint value criteria pattern.

It might be worth emphasizing that in the selection or development of strategies one must not think that rational value analyses in general and the identifying and reducing activities in particular will necessarily result in the resolution of a value conflict (as seen in the resolution attempt in Meux et al. on the legalization of abortion[12]). The action being evaluated may be a disvalue or value conflict action. What the rational value analysis does is provide a way of judging the true value of an action for the participants or—less controversially—provide a value judgment that is not likely to change even after more value analysis activities are undertaken. The closer the judgment to the true value of an action for the participants, the easier to classify an action as a resolution action. Also, given a value conflict on an action, the best way to resolve it on *that* action is by identifying and reducing differences rationally.

Following is a seven-step procedure based on value-highlighting formulation. The first three steps involve a formulation phase—identifying the important sources of conflict and determining where these sources are considered as differences in the subsidiary value judgments. The last four steps involve a resolution phase—some activities are aimed more directly at reducing the differences. The procedure is described for only two participants and is illustrated with the reconstruction of the gun control example.

Step 1. The participants arrive at the session with the value-highlighting fact-assembly charts completed and the values ranked. Each participant examines the other's chart. (See Applegate and Evans for many practical suggestions for performing rational value analyses in general and fact-assembly charts—there called fact-organization charts—in particular.[11])

Figure 1 presents the reconstructed fact-assembly charts for Dee and John. Differences between the participants in their subsidiary value judgments or value realization patterns are assumed to be the main sources of the value conflict.

Step 2. The participants identify important differences in their subsidiary value judgments (i.e., for those values having opposing subsidiary value judgments). Each value on which subsidiary value judgments are not opposing is dropped from further consideration, since it is assumed not to be a source of the value conflict.

Important differences between Dee and John are in the values of freedom, life and legality (especially effectiveness): (1) Dee judges current gun control laws to be infringing on freedom, whereas John judges them to be only somewhat threatening and whatever infringement exists to be necessary; (2) Dee judges the current gun control laws to be ineffective in saving life, whereas John judges them to be highly effective; and (3) Dee judges the current gun control laws to be ineffective *as laws* (as we also saw in the passage saying there are 128 laws being considered in Congress), whereas John judges them to be somewhat effective. Differences on these three values are the most important sources of value conflict, the other important sources being the ranking of values.

Step 3. Participants classify each important difference in subsidiary value judgments into one of three types. In the first type the values are ranked high by both participants; in the second type a value is ranked high by one participant but not by the other participant; in the third type a value is ranked low by both participants. Differences of the third type are dropped from further consideration, since they are not an important source of the value conflict.

In the gun control example there are no differences of the first kind. All differences are of the second kind, except for cost.

Since this is a difference of the third kind, it is dropped from further consideration.

Step 4. This step begins the resolution phase activities. For each of the most important subsidiary value judgments of the first kind, participants simultaneously (1) identify differences in the factual claims assembled in the fact-assembly charts and attempt to reduce differences in both *which* factual claims are retained, added or deleted and in the *quality* or adequacy of evidence of the factual claims; and (2) maintain and even improve the extent to which each participant individually meets the standards of rationality. For each value, participants then decide whether they agreed on the subsidiary value judgment or at least have only an unimportant difference.

In the gun control example there were no differences of the first kind, so this step would not be performed.

Step 5. Repeat the activities in step 4, focusing now on values with differences of the second kind (from step 3).

As already indicated, in the gun control example the participants spent a great deal of effort on these tasks, but it was not organized by the values to which the factual claims were relevant. (Some agreement did take place, however.)

Step 6. For those values of the first and second kind in which subsidiary value judgments still differ importantly, the participants review differences in their rankings of the values to see if the preceding discussion might lead one or both participants to change their rankings. For example, one result might be that a value is viewed as unimportant for both participants, making the difference in subsidiary value judgments a difference of the third kind and thus no longer a source of the value conflict.

In the gun control example there was a brief spontaneous review of this kind, but it did not result in any important changes in rankings of values.

Step 7. At this point the initial incompatible action is not likely to be a resolution action. Thus participants should try other actions—whether existing or new—that seem more likely to be resolution actions. One way would be to produce another action by noting the "negative facts" in the highly ranked values for both participants and trying to modify these characteristics to produce another action better meeting the value criteria pattern.

This is essentially what took place when Dee and John began to agree on the importance of eliminating "Saturday Night Specials" and requiring some type of education in the wise use of guns. In the following passage Dee and John formulate their final value judgments:

Moderator: OK. We're going to conclude now with final value judgments. Dee, what do you have?

Dee: A gun control law that would establish an education program to lower accidents and gun control that would outlaw "Saturday Night Specials" but not interfere with my constitutional right would be desirable.

Moderator: That comes close to a value principle, which is another way of saying

that you kind of specify the characteristics of your gun control law. That's good. OK. John, what do you have?

John: Well, for me I'd still like to see guns out of the hands of the public. I understand that it's not practical to do that and we haven't reached a solution to do that. So for me a training program would be very good in which people who purchase guns would go through a training program and learn safe ways of dealing with guns. I would value that.

Moderator: OK.

John: I'm not sure that's a value judgment.

Moderator: That's pretty close to what we're thinking of as a value judgment. You spelled out characteristics of a gun control law, that it would involve training programs, etc.

John: We still haven't resolved the issue of guns in the hands of the public. Guns at home.

Moderator: Right. That would be, then, if we looked at specific characteristics of a gun control law, there would be some on which you two would have agreement, and then some on which there would still be disagreement. But that's considerable progress over the position we started with.

HEALTH IMPLICATIONS

What if participants in a value conflict situation used this conceptualization as a guide for resolving the value conflict? What beneficial effects, if any, would there be on the participants' health? There seem to be many ways the use of this conceptualization by participants in a value conflict might affect health. For example, impressionistic observations from our own resolution suggest that the use of the conceptualization reduces stress and hostility, helps an individual understand and appreciate both himself or herself and the other (see Meux et al.[12]), and improves an individual's sense of coherence of important aspects of the situation, especially by using the fact-assembly charts. It also seems plausible that there might be increased feelings of self-confidence from being able to cope with both the tactical and strategic aspects of a difficult and complex problem, with an enhanced sense of agency from more rational control over the environment and increased self-control and self-direction from the rational self-legislation. In fact, this conceptualization could readily be viewed as a coping strategy for value conflict; that is, an overall plan of action for overcoming stressors that has the characteristics of rationality, flexibility and farsightedness.[25(p112-113)]

Further support for the plausibility of claims about beneficial effects from using this conceptualization could be obtained by discussing how participants could or might improve on each of Bower's five dimensions of ego processes,[26] by discussing how participants could improve on most of Jahoda's proposed six criteria for mental health as discussed by Loevinger,[27] or by examining implications of the fact that one of the conceptualization's central concepts, the self, is a holistic concept and thus provides a prima facie plausibility for implications for holistic health.

However, only implications of the conceptualization for one important aspect of holistic health, improving a participant's sense of coherence, are focused on here. Antonovsky has recently argued that a person's sense of coherence is one of the central factors, if not *the* central factor, in maintenance of a person's health.[25]

The basic assumption here is that a participant's sense of coherence can be improved by improving the actual coherence of his or her formulations of various aspects of content in the self as object (perceptions, meanings, beliefs, values, and so on). Two kinds of operations are important in improving coherence: clarifying and modifying. Clarifying operations are helpful in improving coherence because they help pinpoint where the lack of coherence exists. Modifying operations increase coherence directly.

Clarifying Existing Coherence

A number of clarifying operations can help participants determine existing coherence. For example, a participant can examine his or her value analysis in the fact-assembly chart to clarify the extent of its coherence—how he or she balances the positive and negative facts for each subsidiary value judgment, ranks the values, and "synthesizes" the subsidiary value judgments into the overall value judgment. When the two participants compare their fact-assembly charts, this will indicate roughly the relative coherence of each participant.

Coherence may also be clarified by examining consistency, since a lack of consistency reduces coherence. For example, a participant may notice that the value rankings in the fact-assembly chart are not consistent with rankings in similar situations, or that some important values to himself or herself have been omitted that have been included in similar situations. The use of the tests for the consistency of a value principle—the new cases test and the subsumption test[5,10,11,18]—may indicate lack of consistency.

Although a formulation can be viewed as clarifying what the coherence is, a formulation may also increase coherence. For example, the formulation of a fact-assembly chart enables a participant to see aspects of the situation "as a whole" and to see relations that are more difficult to grasp in the context of a discussion. This is especially true of conceptual relations, as in the syllogistic kind of reasoning, in the criterion (major premise) and fact (minor premise) together supporting a value judgment (conclusion).[28]

Increasing Coherence

Some modifying operations increase coherence, including balancing, subsuming, reranking, reconceptualizing, reformulating and integrating. One way of increasing coherence is by reformulating the value principle after adding new facts.[11,18] Another way of increasing coherence is by reconceptualizing some aspects of the situation in terms of some conceptualization from psychology or the social sciences, showing how these aspects "hang together" in a way not before considered by the participants.

The reduction of complexity increases coherence, as evidenced in the formulation of a fact-assembly chart.[10] A participant can see the relations of facts to each other in a fact-assembly chart (e.g., how specific facts help warrant general facts), how the facts relate to the values to which they are relevant, that each subsidiary value judgment helps reduce complexity by organizing everything relevant to that value perspective, and how the subsidiary value judgments can be "synthesized" into the overall value judgment. Further, when the two participants study each other's fact-assembly chart, complexity is reduced and thus coherence is increased. Each participant can see what facts are relevant and most important to the other participant, how the values are ranked, and in general see the similarities and differences as a whole.

REFERENCES

1. Werkmeister, W.H. *Man and His Values* (Lincoln, Neb.: University of Nebraska Press 1967).
2. Parker, D.H. *The Philosophy of Value* (Ann Arbor, Mich.: University of Michigan Press 1957).
3. Diggory, J.C. *Self-Evaluation* (New York: John Wiley and Sons, Inc. 1966).
4. Smith, M.B. "Perspectives on Selfhood." *Am Psychol* 33:12 (December 1978) p. 1053-1063.
5. Coombs, J. "Objectives of Value Analysis," in Metcalf, L., ed. *Values Education: Rationale, Strategies, and Procedures* in the 41st Yearbook of the National Council for the Social Studies (Washington, D.C.: National Council for the Social Studies 1971) p. 1-28.
6. Deutsch, M. *The Resolution of Conflict* (New Haven, Conn.: Yale University Press 1973).

7. Nye, R.D. *Conflict Among Humans* (New York: Springer Publishing Co. 1973).
8. Johnson, D.W. and Johnson, R.T."Conflict in the Classroom: Controversy and Learning." *Revue of Educational Research* 49:1 (Winter 1979) p. 51-69.
9. Nagel, T. *Mortal Questions* (Cambridge University Press 1979).
10. Coombs, J. "Teaching Strategies for Value Analysis," in Metcalf, L., ed. *Values Education: Rationale, Strategies, and Procedures* in the 41st Yearbook of the National Council for the Social Studies (Washington, D.C.: National Council for the Social Studies 1971) p. 29-74.
11. Applegate, T. and Evans, K. *Making Rational Decisions* (Salt Lake City: Concept Development, Inc. 1979).

12. Meux, M. "Resolving Value Conflicts," in Metcalf, L., ed. *Values Education: Rationale, Strategies, and Procedures* in the 41st Yearbook of the National Council for the Social Studies (Washington, D.C.: National Council for the Social Studies 1971) p. 120–166.

13. Meux, M, Evans, K. and Applegate, T. *The Development of a Value Observation System for Group Discussion in Decision Making.* Final report of U.S. Office of Education Project No. 0-H-028. (Salt Lake City: Bureau of Educational Research, University of Utah 1972).

14. Edel, A. *Ethical Judgment* (New York: Free Press 1955).

15. Rescher, N. *Introduction to Value Theory* (Englewood Cliffs, N.J.: Prentice-Hall 1969).

16. Taylor, P. *Normative Discourse* (Englewood Cliffs, N.J.: Prentice-Hall 1961).

17. Oliver, D. and Shaver, J. *Teaching Public Issues in the High School* (Boston: Houghton-Mifflin 1966).

18. Evans, K. and Applegate, T. "Value Decisions and the Acceptability of Value Principles." *Values Concepts and Techniques* (Washington, D.C.: National Education Association Publication 1976) p. 148–158.

19. Fisher, R. "Fractionating Conflict," in Fisher, R., ed. *International Conflict and Behavioral Science: The Craigville Papers* (New York: Basic Books 1964).

20. Frost, J. and Wilmot, W. *Interpersonal Conflict* (Dubuque, Iowa: Wm. C. Brown 1978).

21. Meux, M. "A Perspective on Axiological Adequacy—Some Implications for Values Education: Comments on Howard Kirschenbaum's Paper." *The Value Theorists' Approach to Moral/Citizenship Education* presented at the Moral/Citizenship Education Conference, Philadelphia, 1976. (Philadelphia: Research for Better Schools 1978) p. 45–64.

22. Tucker, R. "Assessing Adequacy in Moral Value Change," in Proceedings of the Eighth International Interdisciplinary Conference on Piagetian Theory. (Los Angeles: University of Southern California Press 1979).

23. Edel, A. *Science and the Structure of Ethics* (Chicago: International Encyclopedia of Unified Science 2:3, University of Chicago Press 1961).

24. Edel, A. *Method in Ethical Theory* (New York: Bobbs-Merrill 1963).

25. Antonovsky, A. *Health, Stress, and Coping* (San Francisco: Jossey-Bass 1979).

26. Bower, E. "The Confluence of the Three Rivers—Ego Processes," in Bower, E., ed. *Behavioral Science Frontiers in Education* (New York: John Wiley and Sons 1967) p. 48–71.

27. Loevinger, J. *Ego Development* (San Francisco: Jossey-Bass 1976).

28. Meux, M. and Chadwick, J. "Procedures in Value Analysis," in Metcalf, L., ed. *Values Education: Rationale, Strategies, and Procedures* in the 41st Yearbook of the National Council for the Social Studies (Washington, D.C.: National Council for the Social Studies 1971) p. 75–119.

The Role of Discussion in Ethics Training

Marvin W. Berkowitz, Ph.D.
Assistant Professor of Psychology
Marquette University
Milwaukee, Wisconsin

WHILE THE FIELD of nursing has become aware of the concern for ethics and ethics education for nurses there is still a major flaw with the typical approach to nursing ethics education. This flaw is the consistent lack of concern for the developmental nature of moral thinking, and for the implications of such a concern for prescriptions for nursing education. This flaw must be addressed if nurses are to gain the skills and knowledge necessary to make mature ethical decisions in nursing practice.

EDUCATIONAL PRESCRIPTIONS IN THE NURSING LITERATURE

Many educational prescriptions currently being offered in the nursing literature call for formal ethical training in ethical theory or critical thinking methods. Fromer endorses a case analysis approach to ethics education, but only after discounting her preference for a course taught by a philosopher or nurse-philosopher as impractical in contemporary nursing situations.[1] Whether it is impractical or not, it is certainly not the norm according to Aroskar who points out that only 6 of the 86 baccalaureate nursing programs she surveyed have faculty who "spend half or more of their time teaching ethics." None "had a faculty member with the term 'ethics' in his academic title."[2] Rabb prescribes a more general exposure to moral issues and ethical theories.[3]

Langham, largely in reaction to Rabb, suggests that nurses tend to assume that they already have the answers to moral problems and really make moral decisions on the relatively inappropriate and inefficient basis of intuition.[4] The *Nursing '74* survey of over 1,600 nurses offers tangential support for Langham's assumption by pointing out that two-thirds of nurses feel that their standards are more exacting than those of other nurses, a statistic that is logically impossible.[5] Furthermore, 99 percent of nurses feel that their standards are equal to (72 percent) or greater than (27 percent) those of the physicians they work with. About two-thirds of them also feel "moderately" or "very" sure of themselves.

Nevertheless, although nurses often report theft of hospital supplies and "doctoring" of medical notes as prevalent, they do not apply principles of "blowing the whistle" uniformly to fellow nurses and physicians. This apparent discrepancy in self-perception becomes more problematic when one also considers that 54 percent of the nurses surveyed reported that they would not "call a code" on a terminal patient during an unexpected cardiac arrest when the physician had left no instructions. Langham's concern seems to have

some support, although Langham engages more in moral phenomenology than in empirical investigation and therefore offers no factual support himself. Both his analysis and his subsequent prescription to "produce a neurosis" in students have been rejected by Curtin as inaccurate and therefore inappropriate.[6] We are therefore left without a clear consensus on the issue. Curtin and Langham do agree, however, that ethics education should focus on the training of critical thinking.

A number of authors argue that ethics education must teach nursing students ethical principles and methods. As already noted, Andrews and Hutchinson, Fromer, and Rabb recommend the teaching of certain ethical principles.[7-9] Langham considers self-doubt, or an awareness of ethical relativism, as a necessary first condition for nurses to be able to engage in ethical practice.[10] Shapiro considers altruism to be a necessary but insufficient condition as an ethical motivator for nurses. He states that "nurses' work must be its own reward."[11] Burgess, on the other hand, argues that the personal development of the student nurse should be the rubric for all of nursing education, but unfortunately he offers little in the way of procedures or methods.[12] Rabb suggests that all nurses should be Kantian moralists, a position not incompatible with Stenberg's call for a covenantal basis for nursing practice—a basis which entails a mutual, reciprocal, humanistic and nurturant relationship between patient and health care professional.[13]

Other authors offer a variety of "ethical thinking" or "critical analysis" models. Ryden suggests that a nurse in a moral dilemma ought to evaluate different options on the basis of their merits, but neglects to suggest how such decisions may be made.[14] Bergman offers an eight-step process for making ethical decisions because "ethical decisions are primarily a cognitive process and should be taught in nursing education programmes at all levels."[15] Her method of teaching this in the classroom is simply to engage in class discussions of ethical issues.

Andrews and Hutchinson propose that the successful analysis of a moral dilemma depends on the consideration of evidence.[16] Ironically, these authors offer no evidence for their prescriptions and never mention the variety of authors who have spent their careers studying such moral communications.[17,18] Curtin presents a model of critical ethical analysis that highlights the nurse's individual prolonged grappling with a moral issue, but in a quite contradictory fashion concludes by arguing for the autonomy of the patient in ethical decisions.[19]

These models of ethics education clearly are well intentioned and often quite scholarly, but fall short of practicality for nurs-

---

Current models of ethics education clearly are well intentioned and often quite scholarly, but fall short of practicality for nursing education.

---

ing education. Before a more practical prescription for nursing ethics and education can be established, two key issues that arise in the literature must be examined. The first is a prevalently voiced concern; the second is important for its relative absence in the literature.

TWO CENTRAL ISSUES IN NURSING ETHICS

The first issue concerns the inherently social nature of nursing practice. While this is not a unanimous concern, it has nevertheless been quite frequently linked to problems in nursing ethics. Rabb is perhaps clearest on this issue. Using Buber's terminology, he describes the nurse–client relationship as either I-thou, where the client is regarded as a subjective being conscious of his personhood and suffering, or as I-it, where the client is viewed as an object. In this vein, Rabb argues that "To treat another as a 'thou,' and not merely an 'it,' one must affirm not only the other's self-consciousness, but also his ultimate, irreducible freedom, his autonomy, his self-control."[20] The goal of ethics education, in Rabb's view, is to make the nurse aware of the patient as a subjective being in existential crisis.

In a somewhat more complex fashion, Stenberg also describes the nurse's role as essentially social, involved in a triadic relationship, which interfaces with the physician on the one hand and the patient on the other:

It is the single most important element contributing to the unusual conflicts of nursing practice. . . . At one and the same time, the nurse is expected to function as the agent of the physician, the practitioner of her own profession, and an advocate for the patient.[21]

Stenberg argues further for the "team concept of health delivery" and claims that if "it is to become a reality, nursing and medicine will need to develop a commonality of ethical thought and practice in order to function effectively."[22]

Ryden and Curtin each appear to be somewhat inconsistent on this point.[23,24] Both argue first for a process of *individual* ethical decision making, and then conclude that the dilemma and choice are really the patient's, or, at best, jointly the nurse's and the patient's. The nurse must merely facilitate the patient's decision or perhaps share in it. Others have touched on this issue somewhat indirectly by focusing on social discussion and problem-solving formats for nursing ethics education.[25-27]

It seems that the inherently social nature of nursing practice and, more specifically, nursing ethics is a key aspect of any plan for the ethics training of nurses. What is needed is a sound theoretical rationale and a prescription for educational implementation of such a perspective. This point leads us to the second central issue in the nursing ethics literature which is actually a case of omission.

The developmental level of nurses is neglected in the literature. Only in the past three years has any mention been made of moral development in the literature, and such mention is found in only seven references. Rabb's suggestion that nurses ought to endorse Kantian moral imperatives flies in the face of over 20 years of research concerning the development of moral reasoning capacities.[28] Curtin, outside of those directly endorsing developmental theory, comes closest to acknowledging human development when she argues that:

moral certitude is a characteristic of, although by no means confined to, very young persons. Most students, including nursing students, are very young, thus the emphasis on this particular aspect of teaching—particularly the teaching of ethics.[29]

It is surprising that this emphasis on human development and growth is not more evident in the literature. Nursing as a profession has long emphasized professional development. In addition, the short-term growth of an individual patient is a central concern of nursing. The entire field of teaching, including nursing education, is dedicated not only to the transmission of knowledge but to the development of students as well.[30] Nevertheless, only very recently have a few articles and doctoral dissertations begun to address themselves to the issue of human development in nursing ethics. Even so, little of this work has applied the notion of moral development (the interface of ethics and human development) to the practice of ethical training in nursing curricula.

THE DEVELOPMENTAL APPROACH TO ETHICS EDUCATION

Two basic assumptions can be derived from the two issues discussed above:
- *Assumption one:* The practice of nursing, and therefore the ethical concerns of nursing practice, are essentially social in nature.
- *Assumption two:* The capacity for both social and ethical understanding is developmental in nature.

When Curtin notes the youthful tendency for moral certitude, she is actually observing what developmental psychologists consider a product of adolescent development. This may indeed be what Rabb considers moral egoism.[31] Perry has charted the course of intellectual and ethical understanding in the college years and asserts that the college educator's goal is to help the student move beyond an understanding of the world in which every question has an absolute right answer.[32] Perry terms this world view "dualism." A dualistic world view is common among undergraduate nursing students and often impedes learning. For example, protestations over ambiguous test questions are symptomatic of a view that all knowledge is "black and white" and that ambiguous questions must therefore simply be poorly worded. It is literally *unthinkable* that they could accurately reflect the nature of knowledge.

This capsulization of one developmental concern in nursing education illustrates how developmental psychology can inform nursing education. Traditionally nursing educators would try to remedy a pervasive dualism by trying to *teach* nursing students that knowledge is not absolute. This, however, is a futile practice. To instill an equally pervasive sense of the "relativism" of knowledge (as Perry terms it), one must be sensitive to the developmental underpinnings of such an acquisition. These underpinnings are the very basic tenets of what is called variously the cognitive-developmental model of development, the structural model of development or the stage model of development.[33] Furthermore, when students do reach a stage of relativism, developmental theory again offers the means to move beyond this world view to a new, more mature and effective way of understanding.

This concept of development comes out of a tradition in psychology[34-36] and education[37] that describes the movement of the human organism through a universal and invariant sequence of ways (stages) of understanding the ethical (or any other) world. It is a process of ontogenetic evolution, with each meaning-making system (or stage) that develops subsuming the preceding one, yet being qualitatively different from, and more adequate than, its developmental predecessor.

The individual moves through this developmental process as a product of the interaction of environmental experience with inherent regulatory mechanisms (largely parallel to those of biological and ecological systems). It is a natural and deliberate process. More importantly, it describes a pervasive shift. Movement to a new stage entails the construction of a new general world view. It is not merely a new rule or fact that one acquires, but a whole new way of understanding. Thus it must be developed rather than taught. Perhaps Kegan describes this evolutionary phenomenon best when he rather poetically says, "This evolutionary motion is *the prior*, or *grounding phenomenon. . .;* this process or activity, this adaptive conversation, is the very source of and unifying context for, thought and feeling."[38]

It seems inappropriate to consider a semester course in the philosophy of ethics as sufficient to transform nursing students into Kantian moralists, as Rabb might prescribe.[39] Yet, this seems to be the aim of many contemporary nursing ethics curricula.

Instead it is necessary to look to the

It seems inappropriate to consider a semester course in the philosophy of ethics as sufficient to transform nursing students into Kantian moralists.

theoretical assumptions of this model of human development if one is to usefully create an ethics curriculum for nursing students. This literature suggests that ethical reasoning has an invariant and universal nature and path which may nevertheless be facilitated, remediated or accelerated, but only within limits. As almost 15 years of research in education and psychology have demonstrated, ethics education needs to be structured in certain specific ways if it is to optimally impact on the student's level of ethical reasoning, and even then there is limited room for growth, acceleration or remediation.[40] First, let us examine more precisely what is meant by moral development. (In the psychology and education literatures, the term *moral* is used in lieu of *ethical*. Here the terms are used interchangeably.)

Kohlberg defines morality developmentally as the process of reasoning about issues of justice and fairness.[41] He has demonstrated that this reasoning develops in a series of stages in each individual.[42] These stages, as described above, are universal and invariantly sequenced with each new stage subsuming and surpassing the preceding stage. It is a slow developmental process with most people not reaching the fourth stage until late adolescence (if they reach it at all).

Although Rabb and others suggest that nurses should be *taught* to be Kantian moralists, very few people *develop* such a level of moral thinking and, if they should, rarely before their mid to late 20s at the earliest.[43] Most nursing students will be at a stage of morality typified by concerns with the right and just as determined by maintenance of relationships, conformity and social expectations, and the affective states of affected parties (Stage 3). Many may also be at or moving toward an understanding of the right and just as defined by societally derived obligations, duties and responsibilities and the consequences of an action upon the stability of the system (Stage 4).

The fifth and sixth stages are characterized by a "prior-to-society" perspective and a recognition of universal ethical principles. As noted above, this is largely unknown to undergraduates. Indeed only approximately 10 to 15 percent of adults ever develop any Stage 5 reasoning. Much fewer develop it as a predominant basis for ethical thinking. Nursing ethics curricula should therefore be tailored to initiate and consolidate Stages 3 and 4, not, as Rabb would inappropriately ask, Stages 5 and 6.

It should be pointed out that we are dealing here predominantly with reasoning capacity. There is no guarantee that any individual is going to act on the product of such reasoning. Nevertheless, the development of a more moral stage of reasoning provides the *potential* for, and has been clearly shown to be related to, more moral action.[44]

DEVELOPMENTAL MORAL EDUCATION AND THE NURSING CURRICULUM

As noted earlier, only seven references have been identified that address both moral development and nursing. Of these, four were descriptive studies and three were educational interventions. All the studies reported utilized Rest's Defining Issues Test (DIT),[45] an objective and quicker version of Kohlberg's Moral Judgment Interview (MJI), or a measure of their own. The descriptions of nurses' moral development reveal that nurses seem to be conventional moral reasoners (i.e., at Stages 3 and 4). However, these studies used the DIT which scores an individual approximately one to two stages higher than does the MJI. Furthermore, the DIT measures the level of *preference* for and *recognition* of presented moral reasoning. The MJI assesses one's level of spontaneous *production* of moral reasoning.

Munhall, for instance, is interested in finding the levels of moral reasoning that nurses use in analyzing moral issues.[46] If one assumes that nurses do so by choosing between a smorgasbord of presented pro and con arguments, then the DIT is most appropriate. If, on the other hand, one assumes that nurses make moral decisions by generating their own moral position, a seemingly more veridical position, the MJI is the more appropriate measure of such a capacity. Munhall nonetheless uses the DIT. Schoenrock uses the DIT and finds few nurse practitioners or students beyond the conventional level of moral reasoning.[47] Crisham reports that both familiarity with the content of a dilemma and education are positively related to DIT or DIT-like moral reasoning.[48]

When Kohlberg's stages are presented in the literature, they are as likely to be misrepresented as they are to be accurate.[49,50] Outdated references and information abound. Ketefian, however, offers an accurate and up-to-date summary of Kohlberg moral development and education.[51]

Educational strategies are a prevalent concern in the nursing literature. Many suggestions have been offered, often adopted or adapted from the moral education literature. Some applications have been attempted, with mixed results. Mahon and Fowler used a brief "ethics rounds" intervention with nursing students and found significant moral development to result.[52] Bridston, however, used a similar approach and found no effect.[53] Krawczyk and Kudzma describe a parallel intervention but offer no assessment of its effectiveness.[54] Others have reported a tendency for such programs to be overly informally designed and unstructured. Schoenrock found that nurses perceive themselves as lacking the teaching strategies necessary for moral education.[55] As noted above, Aroskar described a similar weakness in nursing education.[56]

The educational prescriptions offered in the literature have been for Kohlberg's two predominant modes of moral education, classroom discussion and institutional atmosphere or "just community."[57] The latter is more ambitious and probably beyond the practical interest of most of the readers. This article is therefore limited to a treatment of the classroom discussion format.

The nursing literature on Kohlberg moral discussion is similar to the general moral education literature in that it misses one crucial point of moral discussion: individual discussion skills.[58] For instance, in the best treatments of moral discussion in the nursing literature, Ketefian, and Krawczyk and Kudzma recognize the complexity of moral discussion, but never fully develop its features.[59,60]

KOHLBERG MORAL DISCUSSION

Moral discussion dates back to the late 1960s when Kohlberg and his students began classroom and prison interventions in an attempt to accelerate individual moral development. Encouraging results led to an explosive proliferation of books and articles about moral discussion in the 1970s, a trend that continues today. The main features of moral discussion are the following:

1. the topic of discussion must be *moral,* preferably in the form of open-ended dilemmas;
2. *reasoning* about moral issues must be presented, rather than just choices or behavioral solutions;
3. reasoning must include *justifications* for moral prescriptions (i.e., what *ought* to be done);
4. there must be an atmosphere of *openness and acceptance* of others' moral reasoning;
5. there should be a *mixture* of levels of moral reasoning represented in the discussion group;
6. discussants must *confront* each other's moral arguments; and
7. discussants should be exposed to *higher stage reasoning.*

There are two typical confusions about this list. First, item 7 is often interpreted as mandatory and as implying that the facilitator, typically the classroom teacher, must present arguments above the reasoning level of the discussants. While it certainly may enhance such a curriculum, it is not at all necessary for successful moral education.[61] Indeed it is often impractical to expect that sophisticated a command of Kohlberg's stages in a moral discussion facilitator. The second problem has already been alluded to. This is the general neglect of moral discussion skills.

MORAL DISCUSSION SKILLS

Various writers have detailed how to create and direct a moral discussion curriculum (see Galbraith and Jones[62] or Hersh, Paolitto and Reimer[63] for excellent treatments of moral discussion). These authors focus on teacher skills and/or classroom structure and composition. Rarely is any mention made of student training. Nevertheless, it has been demonstrated that the form of discussion used by discussants is significantly related to the effectiveness of the discussion intervention.[64-66] A particular form of moral discussion skills has been

---

Transactive discussion skills have been identified as most likely present in those moral discussions that lead to the moral development of the discussants.

---

identified as most likely to be present in those moral discussions that lead to the development of the discussants. This is called *transactive discussion.* It has been defined as:

discussion in which each member engages the reasoning of his/her discussion partners with his/her own reasoning. Rather than merely providing consecutive assertions, discussants "operate" on each other's reasoning. In a very dialectical sense, one's own reasoning confronts the other's antithetical reasoning in an ongoing dialogic dynamic.[67]

Furthermore, it has been determined that simple re-presentations of another's reasoning, as in reflective counseling, are not effective as a moral discussion intervention form.[68,69] Instead discussants should be more actively analyzing and transforming both their own and their co-discussants' reasoning about moral issues.

Why does transactive discussion lead to more development? Simply because it is more likely to produce what is called *cognitive conflict* or *disequilibrium*. This concept is central to stage theory. One is expected to develop to the next stage only when the following two conditions exist: (1) the present stage is completed and consolidated, and (2) disconfirming experiences have led to a questioning of the present stage and a resultant experience of cognitive conflict or disequilibrium. Transactive discussion, especially the transformational form, is likely to provide more of those disconfirming experiences by centering around the analysis and comparison of moral arguments with an eye toward the adequacy of such arguments for resolving moral problems.

THE TRANSACTIVE MODEL

Thus far 18 categories of transactive behavior have been identified, of which 6 are of the lower order reflective type and 12 are of the higher order transformational type. The former are called *Representational* and the latter *Operational*. All categories (and individual transactive speech acts) are called *Transacts*. As noted above, only Operational Transacts are empirically related to successful (development-producing) moral discussions. The role of the Representational Transacts is not yet clearly understood, but it seems that they serve to facilitate discussion while not actually facilitating the development of moral reasoning.

Representational Transacts

There are only four pure Representational Transacts (see Table 1). Included in the category are two other Transacts that are neither Representational nor Operational. These are called Elicitational, and they are simply requests for information. One, called *Feedback Request*, is a request for confirmation of understanding and/or agreement by the discussion partner. The other, *Justification Request*, is a request for another to justify his or her moral argument.

The Representational Transacts are relatively passive re-presentations of another's moral reasoning. The classic case, *Paraphrase*, is a simple nonverbatim recapitulation of another's reasoning, much like a counselor's reflective response. Note that no conceptual transformation (rather simply a linguistic transformation) is being performed in such an act. The stage and nature of the argument remain unaltered.

The other Representational Transacts are *Juxtaposition, Dyad Paraphrase* and *Competitive Juxtaposition*. The first is a simple case of consecutive paraphrases of one's own argument and that of one or more others. The last is actually a variation of the first. Competitive Juxtaposition entails a juxtaposition with a valuing statement that indicates which parts of each person's argument are accepted or rejected by the speaker. Dyad Paraphrase is a Transact in which the speaker is recapitulating a shared moral argument rather than the separate arguments of different individuals. One

Table 1. Formal Transacts

Primary Focus	Noncompetitive mode	Competitive mode
Ego	**Feedback Request (E)** Do you understand or agree with my position? **Clarification (O)** (a) No, what I am trying to say is the following. (b) Here's a clarification of my position to aid in your understanding.	**Competitive Clarification (O)** My position is not necessarily what you take it to be. **Refinement (O)** (a) I must refine my position or point as a concession to your position or point (subordinative mode). (b) I can elaborate or qualify my position to defend against your critique (super-ordinative mode).
Alter	**Paraphrase (R/E)** (a) I can understand and paraphrase your position or reasoning. (b) Is my paraphrase of your reasoning accurate? **Justification Request (E)** Why do you say that? **Completion (R/O)** I can complete or continue your unfinished reasoning. **Extension (O)** (a) Here's a further thought or an elaboration offered in the spirit of your position. (b) Are you implying the following by your reasoning?	**Competitive Paraphrase (R/O)** Here's a paraphrase of your reasoning that highlights its weakness. **Contradiction (O)** There is a logical inconsistency in your reasoning. **Reasoning Critique (O)** (a) Your reasoning misses an important distinction, or involves a superfluous distinction. (b) Your position implicitly involves an assumption that is questionable ("premise attack"). (c) Your reasoning does not necessarily lead to your conclusion/opinion, or your opinion has not been sufficiently justified. (d) Your reasoning applies equally well to the opposite opinion. **Competitive Extension (O)** (a) Would you go to this implausible extreme with your reasoning? (b) Your reasoning can be extended to the following extreme, with which neither of us would agree. **Counter Consideration (O)** Here is a thought or element that cannot be incorporated into your position.
Dyad or Ego/Alter	**Juxtaposition (R)** Your position is x and my position is y. **Common Ground/Integration (O)** (a) We can combine our positions into a common view. (b) Here's a general premise common to both of our positions. **Dyad Paraphrase (R)** Here is a paraphrase of a shared position.	**Competitive Juxtaposition (R)** I will make a concession to your position, but also reaffirm part of my position. **Comparative Critique (O)** (a) Your reasoning is less adequate than mine because it is incompatible with the important consideration here. (b) Your position makes a distinction which is seen as superfluous in light of my position, or misses an important distinction which my position makes. (c) I can analyze your example to show that it does not pose a challenge to my position.

O = Operational.   R = Representational.   E = Elicitational.

can see that all these Transacts are facilitative, but it becomes clear when exploring Operational Transacts that the Representational Transacts are far from ideal at producing cognitive conflict and development.

Operational Transacts

The 12 Operational Transacts share one common feature: they all represent a speaker's transformation and analysis of his or her own or another's moral reasoning in contrast with the partner's (own or other's) reasoning. There are actually two hybrid Transacts (Representational/Operational), but they will be treated as pure Operational Transacts for the sake of this discussion.

In this article, discussion has thus far been limited to dialogues. Therefore, the term Dyad Paraphrase was used above as opposed to Group Paraphrase. There is no reason to believe that what has been learned about moral dialogues is not transferable to larger discussions. In fact, the informal analyses of group moral discussion transcripts reveal a ready application of the Transactive Coding Model to such circumstances. Nonetheless, the current model, as will become clear shortly, is based on a dyadic paradigm.

The 12 Operational Transacts can be divided into three groups, called *Primary Foci*. They refer to whose reasoning is most centrally involved in the speech act. The three types are *Ego* (own reasoning), *Alter* (other's reasoning) and *Dyad* (shared reasoning or equal focus on Ego's and Alter's reasoning). This trichotomy is quite useful in identifying transactive speech acts. Furthermore, each Primary Focus has been divided into two modes of transaction,

Noncompetitive and *Competitive*. The latter transacts are those aimed at "winning" or "losing" an argument. The former are either cooperative or competitively neutral.

Ego-Focus Operational Transacts

Ego-Focus Operational Transacts are moral discussion behaviors that focus primarily on one's own reasoning and entail a transformation or an analysis of reasoning. For a speech act to be transactive it must always involve one's own perspective and that of another. Ego-Focus Transacts are merely more primarily focused on one's own reasoning, but are doing so in the context of, or in response to, the reasoning of another. Likewise, Alter-Focus Transacts are primarily focused on another's reasoning, but are being considered from the vantage point of one's own perspective.

There are two Competitive and one Noncompetitive Ego-Focus Operational Transacts. The Noncompetitive form is called *Clarification*. This represents an attempt to clarify one's own reasoning to improve another's comprehension. The competitive parallel to this is *Competitive Clarification* which describes attempts to disprove or correct another's apparent misunderstanding of one's own reasoning in order to defend one's position. The other Competitive Ego-Focus Transact is called *Refinement*. Here one is not merely clarifying, but is actually altering one's prior reasoning in order either to make a concession to another or to parry another's critique. One should be able to see that all of these Transacts are primarily concerned with one's own reasoning, but that the reasoning of another is always involved, for example, in Refinement it is being defended against.

Alter-Focus Operational Transacts

There are two Noncompetitive and five Competitive Alter-Focus Operational Transacts. The Noncompetitive forms are labeled *Completion* and *Extension*. Completions are simply cases of providing closure to another's unfinished or interrupted moral argument. Extensions are cases of either declarative or interrogative elaborations of another's reasoning.

The five identified Alter-Focus Operational Transacts are all attempts at "winning" the argument by critiquing or defusing another's moral reasoning. The first type, *Competitive Paraphrase*, is a rather subtle and often sarcastic attempt to distortively re-present another's reasoning so as to highlight its weakness. *Contradiction* is a more straightforward pointing out of another's self-contradiction. The third type, and the most prevalent type, is called *Reasoning Critique*. This includes any attempt to demonstrate a flaw in another's reasoning other than by pointing out another's self-contradiction. Reasoning Critiques may take the form of discrediting an underlying premise, of noting a logical flaw in an argument, or of some other criticism. *Competitive Extension*, the fourth type, is composed of statements that challenge another's reasoning by extending it to absurdity. It is as if the speaker is saying "Would you go to this implausible extreme with your reasoning?"

The fifth and final case of Competitive Alter-Focus Transacts is *Counter Consideration*. Here the speaker is setting up a "roadblock" for another's reasoning by offering an idea or example that is anticipated to be problematic by being incompatible with his or her reasoning. In all of the Alter-Focus Transacts one should be able to see that the Primary Focus is the reasoning of another, but analyzed from one's own (Ego's) point of view.

Dyad-Focus Operational Transacts

There are two Dyad-Focus Operational Transacts, one Noncompetitive and one Competitive. The Competitive form is called *Comparative Critique*. It entails demonstrations that another's reasoning is less adequate than one's own reasoning. Note that both perspectives must be overtly considered here. This is what characterizes it as Dyad-Focus. The Noncompetitive form is actually the ideal form of transactive discussion. It is called *Common Ground/Integration*. The more common, and less ideal, version is Common Ground which is simply a presentation of that which one's own reasoning has in common with another's (e.g., identifying a shared premise). The more unusual and ideal version is Integration. Here one is offering an argument that is a synthesis, in a true dialectical sense, of one's own argument and that of another. It represents an attempt to integrate both positions into one mutually acceptable position.

These 18 Transacts are not presented as an exhaustive list. Other Transacts may exist. Also, these Transacts may not do justice to the moral discussions of children. Currently Damon is studying this domain of moral discourse.[70] However, these 18 Transacts can capture the bulk of adolescent and adult moral discourse.

IMPLICATIONS FOR AND APPLICATIONS TO NURSING EDUCATION

The most important question one may ask at this juncture is what all this technical psychological language has to do with nursing. Developmental moral education speaks directly to both key issues given at the beginning of this article, i.e., the social and developmental nature of nursing ethics. Developmental moral education is inherently social, since morality itself is understood as a social phenomenon. Morality is defined as fairness and justice in the *distribution* of goods and rights *among people*. Nursing is always concerned with dilemmas of fairness and justice.

Furthermore, it is important to understand that the moral reasoning of nurses and nursing students is a developmental phenomenon. Therefore, the goal of a nursing ethics education curriculum

---

The goal of a nursing ethics education curriculum should be to nurture the development of higher forms of moral reasoning.

---

should be to nurture the development of higher forms of moral reasoning as well as to consolidate current forms in nursing students. This can be done by following the tenets of developmental moral education as outlined above.

Finally, to be most effective in employing the developmental education model, one must be concerned with the form that moral discussion, the heart of such education, takes. Transactive moral discussion facilitates both moral discussion and the resultant individual development.

Currently, there is no formal training model for transactive discussion skills. However, the following outline of a classroom training procedure is offered:

Step 1: Use videotapes or prepared scripts (available from the author) to present stereotypical transactive and nontransactive dialogues. Have the group discuss the differences between the two dialogues.

Step 2: In a lecture format explain the transactive model and define all the Transacts. Give the students written summaries of the Transacts (a table of Transacts and an 80-page coding manual are also available from the author). Use examples liberally.

Step 3: Pair students and ask them to engage in moral dialogues. They may choose their own moral dilemmas or the teacher may provide them. Instruct students to attempt to use one of the Transacts in the discussion. They should be stopping and processing the discussion whenever they wish in order to plan, forewarn, edit or acknowledge the use of the Transacts. They should also monitor and help each other.

Step 4: Immediately after Step 3, the dyads should be instructed to stop their moral discussions and reflect on how the exercise went (still in their same pairings). Ask them to talk about the degree of difficulty of the talks and about the clarity of the Transacts.

Step 5: Then, and immediately, ask them, still in their pairs, to see if they can remember any Transacts they unintentionally used in Step 4.

Step 6: The whole group should reassemble for clarification and trouble shooting.

All or part of this process can be repeated as frequently as is comfortable for the class and facilitator. It can be interspersed throughout the moral discussion curriculum. Also the instructor should be circulating during the transactive discussion training and offering guidance and support to the student pairs. As time passes, the students should become more familiar and comfortable with transactive

discussion. Then the large group discussions, the body of moral education, will be more likely to produce the desired result—individual moral development.

In closing, it is important to point out that these are not unnatural discussion skills for adolescents and adults. In fact, every one of them was empirically derived from the spontaneous utterances of college students in moral discussions. Operational Transacts alone accounted for about 25 percent of all statements in one study of unguided dyadic discussions of moral dilemmas. Furthermore, none of those students was given any training or special instructions. This training model is merely an attempt to enhance the value of moral discussion by increasing the degree to which it is transactive. If we can achieve this goal in nursing ethics education, we can hope to raise the level of moral decision making of nurses and thereby the opportunity for more moral behavior in nursing practice.

REFERENCES

1. Fromer, M.J. "Teaching Ethics by Case Analysis." *Nursing Outlook* 28 (October 1980) p. 604-609.
2. Aroskar, M.A. "Ethics in the Nursing Curriculum." *Nursing Outlook* 25 (April 1977) p. 260-264.
3. Rabb, J.D. "Implications of Moral and Ethical Issues for Nurses." *Nursing Forum* 15:2 (1976) p. 168-179.
4. Langham, P. "Open Forum: On Teaching Ethics to Nurses." *Nursing Forum* 16:3, 4 (1977) p. 221-227.
5. "Probe." *Nursing '74* (September 1974) p. 35-44.
6. Curtin, L.L. "Nursing Ethics: Theories and Pragmatics." *Nursing Forum* 17:1 (1978) p. 4-11.
7. Andrews, S. and Hutchinson, S.A. "Teaching Nursing Ethics: A Practical Approach." *Journal of Nursing Education* 20:1 (1981) p. 6-11.
8. Fromer. "Teaching Ethics by Case Analysis."
9. Rabb. "Implications of Moral and Ethical Issues."
10. Langham. "Open Forum."
11. Shapiro, B. "The Dead End of Altruism: A Note to Nurses." *Nursing Forum* 15:4 (1976) p. 384-389.
12. Burgess, G. "The Personal Development of the Nursing Student as a Conceptual Framework" *Nursing Forum* 17:1 (1978) p. 96-102.
13. Stenberg, M.J. "The Search for a Conceptual Framework as a Philosophic Basis for Nursing Ethics: An Examination of Code, Contract, Context, and Covenant." *Military Medicine* 144:1 (1979) p. 9-22.
14. Ryden, M.B. "An Approach to Ethical Decision-Making." *Nursing Outlook* 26:11 (1978) p. 705-706.
15. Bergman, R. "Ethics—Concepts and Practice." *International Nursing Review* 20:5 (1973) p. 140-141, 152.
16. Andrews and Hutchinson. "Teaching Nursing Ethics."

17. Argyris, C. and Schon, D.A. *Theory in Practice: Increasing Professional Effectiveness* (San Francisco: Jossey-Bass 1974).
18. Habermas, J. "Moral Development and Ego Identity." *Telos* 24 (Summer 1975), p. 41-55.
19. Curtin, L.L. "A Proposed Model for Critical Ethical Analysis." *Nursing Forum* 17:1 (1978) p. 12-17.
20. Rabb. "Implications of Moral and Ethical Issues." p. 171-172.
21. Stenberg. "The Search for a Conceptual Framework." p. 10-11.
22. Ibid.
23. Ryden. "An Approach to Ethical Decision-Making."
24. Curtin. "A Proposed Model for Critical Ethical Analysis."
25. Bergman. "Ethics—Concepts and Practice."
26. Fromer. "Teaching Ethics by Case Analysis."
27. Andrews and Hutchinson. "Teaching Nursing Ethics."
28. Rabb. "Implications of Moral and Ethical Issues."
29. Curtin. "Nursing Ethics," p. 6.
30. Burgess. "The Personal Development of the Nursing Student."
31. Rabb. "Implications of Moral and Ethical Issues."
32. Perry, W.G., Jr. *Forms of Intellectual and Ethical Development in the College Years: A Scheme.* (New York: Holt, Rinehart and Winston 1970).
33. Kohlberg, L. "Stage and Sequence: The Cognitive-Developmental Approach to Socialization" in Goslin, D.A. (ed.) *Handbook of Socialization Theory and Research.* (Chicago: Rand McNally & Co. 1969) p. 347-480.
34. Baldwin, J.M. *Thought and Things* 3 vols. (London: Swann Sonnenschein, 1906-1911).
35. Kohlberg, L. "Stage and Sequence: The Cognitive-Developmental Approach to Socialization."
36. Piaget, J. *The Moral Judgment of the Child.* Translated by M. Gabain (New York: Free Press 1965).
37. Dewey, J. *Democracy and Education* (New York: Macmillan 1916).
38. Kegan, R.G. "The Evolving Self: A Process Conception for Ego Psychology." *Counseling Psychologist* 8:2 (1979) p. 9.
39. Rabb. "Implications of Moral and Ethical Issues."
40. Lockwood, A.L. "The Effects of Values Clarification and Moral Development Curricula on School-Age Subjects: A Critical Review of Recent Research." *Review of Educational Research* 48:3 (1978) p. 325-364.
41. Kohlberg, L. "Moral Stages and Moralization: The Cognitive-Developmental Approach" in Lickona, T. ed. *Moral Development and Behavior: Theory, Research, and Social Issues.* (New York: Holt, Rinehart and Winston 1976).

42. Kohlberg, L. *The Meaning and Measurement of Moral Development.* Heinz Werner Memorial Lecture, Clark University, Worcester, Mass. 1979.
43. Rabb. "Implications of Moral and Ethical Issues."
44. Kohlberg, L. "The Claim to Moral Adequacy of a Highest Stage of Moral Judgment." *Journal of Philosophy* 70:18 (1973) p. 630-646.
45. Rest, J.R. *Development in Judging Moral Issues* (Minneapolis: University of Minnesota Press 1979).
46. Munhall, P. "Moral Reasoning Levels of Nursing Students and Faculty in a Baccalaureate Nursing Program." *Image* 12:3 (1980) p. 57-61.
47. Schoenrock, N.B. "An Analysis of Moral Reasoning Levels and the Implications for the Nursing Curriculum." *Dissertation Abstracts International* 39:7(1979) p. 4035-A.
48. Crisham, P. "Moral Judgment of Nurses in Hypothetical and Nursing Dilemmas." *Dissertation Abstracts International* 40:9 (1980) p. 4212-B.
49. Krawczyk, R. and Kudzma, E. "Ethics: A Matter of Moral Development." *Nursing Outlook* 26:4(1978) p. 254-257.
50. Mahon, K.A. and Fowler, M.D. "Moral Development and Clinical Decision-Making." *Nursing Clinics of North America* 14:1(1979) p. 3-12.
51. Ketefian, S. "Judging Ethical Issues in Nursing: Research Strategy and Selected Correlates" in Chaska, N. ed. *The Nursing Profession: A Time to Speak* (N.Y.: McGraw-Hill, forthcoming).
52. Mahon and Fowler. "Moral Development and Clinical Decision-Making."
53. Bridston, E.O. "The Development of Principled Moral Reasoning in Baccalaureate Nursing Students." *Dissertation Abstracts International* 40:3(1979) p. 1237-A.
54. Krawczyk and Kudzma. "Ethics: A Matter of Moral Development."
55. Schoenrock. "An Analysis of Moral Reasoning Levels."
56. Aroskar. "Ethics in the Nursing Curriculum."
57. Kohlberg, L. "The Cognitive-Developmental Approach to Moral Education" in Scharf, P. ed. *Reading in Moral Education* (Minneapolis: Winston Press 1978).
58. Berkowitz, M.W. "A Critical Appraisal of the Plus-one Convention in Moral Education." *Phi Delta Kappan* 62:7(1981) p. 488-489.
59. Ketefian. "Judging Ethical Issues in Nursing."
60. Krawczyk and Kudzma. "Ethics: A Matter of Moral Development."
61. Berkowitz. "A Critical Appraisal."
62. Galbraith, R.E. and Jones, T.M. *Moral Reasoning: A Teaching Handbook for Adapting Kohlberg to the Classroom* (Minneapolis: Greenhaven Press 1976).

63. Hersh, R., Paolitto, D. and Reimer, J. *Promoting Moral Growth: From Piaget to Kohlberg* (New York: Longman 1979).

64. Berkowitz, M.W. "The Role of Transactive Discussion in Moral Development: The History of a Six-Year Program of Research-Part I." *Moral Education Forum* 5(Summer 1980) p. 13-26.

65. Berkowitz, M.W. "The Role of Transactive Discussion in Moral Development: The History of a Six-Year Program of Research-Part II." *Moral Education Forum* 5(Fall 1980) p. 15-27.

66. Berkowitz, M.W. and Gibbs, J.C. "Measuring the Developmental Features of Moral Discussion." *Merrill–Palmer Quarterly* 29:4(1983) p. 399-410.

67. Berkowitz, "The Role of Transactive Discussion in Moral Development," p. 13.

68. Berkowitz, M.W. "The Role of Discussion in Moral Education" in Berkowitz, M.W. and Oser, F. eds. *Moral Education: Theory and Application* (Hillsdale, N.J.: L. Erlbaum, 1985).

69. Berkowitz, M.W. and Prestby, J. "Transactive Communication in Peer Counseling." Paper presented at the Eighty-Eighth Annual Convention of the American Psychological Assocaition, Montreal, Canada, September 1980.

70. Damon, W. and Killen, M. "Peer Interaction and the Process of Change in Children's Moral Reasoning." Paper read at the annual meeting of the American Association for the Advancement of Science, Toronto, Canada, January 1981.

The What and How of Ethics Education

Carol Gilbert, Ph.D., R.N.
Chairperson, Undergraduate Division
Associate Professor
Lienhard School of Nursing
Pace University
Pleasantville, New York

HEALTH CARE providers are often faced with ethical dilemmas. With the increasing independent and interdependent functioning of professional nurses, ethical questions surrounding and affecting their delivery of health care are becoming more important and frequent. The evidence in this regard is well documented in the literature.

No longer can nurses deny their accountability and responsibility in the planning and delivery of health care. The fields of anatomy, physiology, pathophysiology, psychology and law can no longer provide consistent solutions to the questions of client need where moral conflict exists. Moreover, Aroskar points out that developments in the sciences often lead the nurse to even more personal and professional moral conflict.[1] The old idea of "do no harm" which has been a hallmark of medicine and nursing is no longer an easy concept to implement.

If one will then accept that the need exists for the inclusion of content concerning ethics and ethical decision making in the nursing curriculum, the question facing nursing would appear to be what type of ethics education should be offered? And, associated with that, how should ethics content be offered?

THE WHAT OF ETHICS EDUCATION

Facilitation of reasoning

It is important to understand at the outset that the terms *ethics* and *morals* are not synonymous. Ethics is "the study of rational processes for determining the best course of action in the face of conflicting choices."[2] Morals refers to "action in accordance to rules of 'right' conduct."[3] Morality, in the sense of a set of culturally defined goals or rules, is more or less external to an individual and imposed on that individual. The goals or rules do not demand reasoning as the basis of agreement on the part of the individual receiving them, even though some reason for the rules may be provided. It is the reasoned use of these goals or rules that comprises ethics, while it is the existence of such goals or rules in the individual's repertoire that is the domain of morals.

With this in mind it is clear that the teaching of ethics should be directed toward placing the learner in the "position of being able to decide what he should do in each situation he may be up against; and, for this, it is necessary but not sufficient to teach him the ends or principles involved. We must also supply him with the knowledge required to apply the principles."[4]

The importance of this point cannot be overemphasized. In the past, a lack of

The overall purpose of ethics content is the facilitation of learner reasoning with respect to moral conflict.

appreciation of the difference between the facilitation of learner reasoning in reference to principles or rules (ethics) and learner action because of rules (morals) led many nurse educators, among others, to teach "how to behave" rather than "how to think" in the face of moral conflict. Clearly then, the overall purpose of ethics content is the facilitation of learner reasoning with respect to moral conflict.

Goals for focusing content

However, since the purpose of ethics content as stated above is so broad, it might be helpful to rework it into a more circumscribed framework, a set of goals. The use of goals not only assists in focusing the content; it also serves as a guide for separating content into several courses, if that option is desired.

Callahan presents such a set of goals.[5] Using what appears to be a developmental framework, he suggests the following: (1) stimulating the moral imagination; (2) recognizing ethical issues; (3) eliciting a sense of moral obligation; (4) developing analytical skills; and (5) tolerating—and resisting—disagreement and ambiguity.

Callahan's first goal involves an area that most nursing curricula currently deal with very effectively: values clarification. Clearly, the affective value/moral system of the learner must not be ignored; without adequate consideration of the learner's own value system, students may have considerable difficulty separating the affective from the cognitive. In this context the cognitive domain is referred to in the second goal—recognition of ethical issues. One might describe this recognition as a type of cognitive sorting of the affective or value system of an individual or group.

In goal three Callahan points out the demand relationship of action to ethical decision making, and emphasizes the need to communicate this concept. To discuss ethics in a purely theoretical way is to violate its function, for ethics is a process of decision making that leads to and demands action, not just the suggestion thereof.

Goal four refers to the intellectual rules and principles involved in the reasoning process and the need for skill development in this area. Obviously, if one is to use logical reasoning one must learn the rules of organization.

Finally, the fifth goal identifies one of the most frustrating parts of ethics, the fact that there are no facts, no "rights" or "wrongs." This feature appears to be especially frustrating to professionals. As students, nurses learn to look for the facts, to base decisions on research. They also learn that while implementation of a decision is a matter of style and therefore may vary among nurses, any other professional in the same situation will arrive at the same basic decision. In ethical decision making, facts do not exist, there are no "concretes" to lean on; one is dealing with abstracts. In the same situation two professionals could and often do arrive at different decisions. Thus the frustration. What legitimizes the inclusion of this goal is that knowing from the outset that this frustration will exist appears to help the learner to cope more easily and effectively.

Specific content areas

Values clarification

Using these goals, specific content areas can now be more easily identified. In logical sequence, the first area of content inclusion should be material dealing with personal and professional values clarification. Here is where learners should be assisted to bring their values and moral beliefs to a conscious level. Study of nursing's code of ethics is a helpful tool. Frequently the use of the ANA Code as an outside source enables the learner to more easily identify and verbalize previously unrealized personal beliefs and values. In addition, comparison of personal beliefs about the profession with the code helps learners to more clearly identify their beliefs about the profession. Presentation and discussion of the Patients' Bill of Rights are also suggested. Inclusion of the bill in this area can facilitate identification of areas of confusion and conflict for the learner with respect to the overall health care delivery system, the roles of different professional groups and the client.

Issue identification

Once learners have a basic grasp of their values and those of the profession, content concerning ethical issues or problem identification can be introduced. Concurrently, presentation of the basic definitions and rules governing what ethics is and how one goes about making an ethical decision should be included. Using this knowledge, learners can then be helped to identify ethical issues of professional and personal concern. Which and how many issues are identified depend on relevance to the learners, time allocation and perhaps the goals of the nursing program. It is very easy to get "bogged down" at this point in endless affective type debate about the issues raised. Because content concerning issue analysis and the decision-making process has yet to be presented in detail, extensive debate of issues is best deferred until such time as the learners have this knowledge.

Along with issue identification, content concerning the affective sense of moral obligation (the need to act on ethical decisions) should be introduced. By offering this material concurrently, learners should be able to more easily begin appreciating the demand relationship between problem identification, decision making and action.

Basic ethical theory

The next content package should logically deal with the analytic phase of ethical decision making. It is at this point that each program designer will have to make decisions concerning depth and breadth of material offered. A solid grounding in normative ethics is essential. Merely defining the concept and presenting a survey of teleology and deontology and one or two decision-making guides derived therefrom, for example, are not sufficient. This superficial approach too often leads learners to assume that ethical decision making is "easy" once one learns the "rules" or "formulas." In addition, if this assumption is made, the serious nature of decision making can be grossly undermined. Works like Brody's *Ethical Decisions in Medicine,*[6] Thompson and Thompson's *Ethics in Nursing,*[7] and Fromer's *Ethical Issues in Healthcare,*[8] while very good, take a less than thorough approach to

ethics theory. They tend to rush the reader through basic ethical theory on the way to discussions of issues. Granted, this is difficult material; however, teaching basic theory is essential if learners are to achieve the ability to "live with" and "act upon" the decisions they make.

Furthermore, the understanding and development of the ability to tolerate and reduce, through the construction of logical arguments, the ambiguity that exists in ethics will be very difficult for the learner. Without this knowledge it would seem unreasonable to expect learners to fully appreciate that ethics has no rights or wrongs and that it is the logic of the decision-making process with its associated justification that is debatable rather than the decision/action. In this regard, material offered in such works as Frankena's *Ethics,*[9] Smart and Williams's *Utilitarianism For and Against,*[10] and Kant's *Groundwork of the Metaphysics of Morals*[11] can be most helpful.

Issue analysis

With knowledge of basic ethical theory learners can then proceed more effectively to the area of issue analysis. The possibility of learners basing decisions on emotion and values rather than on logical reasoning should, at this point, be much less probable. Learners who are able to understand the basic philosophies and then match and adapt them to their personal value systems can more easily redirect their emotional reactions to an issue into a logical reasoning process.

Lest the learner assume that logical reasoning is devoid of affect and therefore mechanical or inhumane, this is a good

Ethics provides individuals with the means to redirect their emotional, illogical reactions . . . into passionate, logically reasoned responses.

time to help learners to understand the difference between emotionalism and passion. Clearly, ethical issues and moral conflicts are human and therefore emotionally loaded. What learners should be helped to appreciate is that ethics does not demand the elimination of the affective response. Rather, ethics provides individuals with the means to redirect their emotional, illogical reactions in the face of moral conflict into passionate, logically reasoned responses. The term passion is used to identify the affective response where it is manifested through reason.

The issues that currently appear to be of most interest to health care professions are those concerning client rights, truth telling, informed consent, rights of human subjects in research, genetic research, and the broad area of quality of life which includes such concerns as euthanasia and abortion. Again, how many and which issues are included in any curriculum should be dependent on learner interest, time allocation and program goals. In addition to those references already mentioned, the *Encyclopedia of Bioethics*[12] is an excellent source for preparation.

Application in professional practice

One final area that is essential in any ethics curriculum is content concerning the application of ethical decision making in professional practice. More specifically,

what is involved in and how does the professional practitioner go about incorporating ethical decision making/action in one's practice?

While this would appear to be a logical question, the problem is that none of the ethics literature currently available really addresses the question. What the literature does is present ethics and ethical decision making from a personal perspective. That is, it assumes that the individual is the unit of ethical decision making. This may be satisfactory on a personal level, but it is quite problematic on a professional level. This is because rarely, if ever, do professional health care providers practice in isolation. While nurses or physicians label clients as "theirs" and say they are autonomous professional practitioners, this is not, strictly speaking, the case. True, one can argue that that which is nursing is autonomous to nurses and that which is medicine is the physician's, but it is also true that there is an ever-expanding area of overlap that is "claimed" by both groups. In addition, it is more usual than rare that the actions of one professional practitioner have implications for, if not direct impact on, another. Granted, some of the professionally oriented ethics literature has reordered this perspective and offers a two-person grouping as the decision-making unit, professional and client, when discussing some professional ethical issues. However, as has been demonstrated above, this is not sufficient.

In professional ethical decision making the unit is not singular or dual; rather it is a triad: professional-client-professional (i.e., nurse-patient-physician). To ignore this reality is to leave the learner with no opportunity to develop strategies for coping with the reality of: "I see your point, Nurse, and understand your ethical position concerning quality of life, but if Mrs. Jones arrests, I order you to initiate resuscitation regardless of what you or the client may have decided." Or "I'm glad I am dealing with a nurse who understands that an ethical conflict exists in this situation. However, I am the client and you must respect my right to decide what is best for me."

While some might argue that this concern is merely a factor to be included in the decision-making process, this is not always so. Granted, consideration of other professional group members and clients could be included in the decision-making process of an individual if they are operating out of some type of teleological framework. However, teleology is not the only existent ethical framework.

Others might say that this triad phenomenon is actually a separate issue. While professional interrelationship can form the basis of an ethical conflict (i.e., autonomy), this contention is too limiting. Rather, the existence of this phenomenon is not only the basis of an issue in and of itself, but it is a factor that is involved in almost every ethical decision in one's professional life. Therefore, it must be given due respect and emphasis. Only in this way can the assumption made by many, that ethics is all well and good in the classroom but just not applicable in the real world, be dealt with effectively.

In this regard, a presentation of and critical discussion about this triad phenomenon should be included in the ethics curriculum. Such a presentation will provide an opportunity for learners to continue developing their appreciation of the importance of using ethical decision making in their practice. Only by redirecting emotion to passion, feeling to committed logic, can professional practitioners hope to help others realize that ethical conflicts exist and that their decisions concerning a conflict are justified, even if not agreed with, and that they cannot be ignored.

Finally, for those considering offering more than just a basic curriculum in ethics, consideration should be given to offering content concerning such concept areas as justice and rights. One might even consider addressing the area of metaphysics.

THE HOW OF ETHICS EDUCATION

When designing the methodology for any specific curriculum content, several things should be considered: the purpose and goals of the content, the learner population, the type of content to be offered and the methodology currently being used for other areas of the curriculum.

In this regard educators should use the small-group seminar with content structured into self-paced modular units divided by goals and arranged using specific behavioral objectives in association with learning activities. In addition, this content should be offered as a separate course rather than integrated throughout the overall curriculum.

The small-group approach is recommended because of the nature and suggested purpose of ethics in nursing education. Clearly, if one is to facilitate the use of reasoning in another individual, the learner must have the opportunity to practice with guidance. The use of small groups also provides the opportunity for learners to maximize their learning by "teaching" each other through discussion and debate. The power of this "teaching effect," first described by Zajonc and Markus,[13] was demonstrated in a recent study on the teaching of ethics.[14] Furthermore, in small groups learners can be more easily helped to cope with the frustrations involved in ethics.

The use of self-paced modular units, based on goals, specific behavioral objectives and learning activities, is an excellent response to the needs of professional nursing students. It not only allows for the fact that people learn at different rates, but it also provides a means of control for learners with respect to other demands on their time. This latter point is an important consideration since a large portion of the nursing student population is in part-time study.

The recommendation that this content be offered as a separate component rather than being integrated throughout the full curriculum stems from the knowledge that writing behavioral objectives in this area, or evaluating student learning, is very difficult. Furthermore, packaging this content as a separate component would mean that it is transferable, not only within a curriculum but physically. That is, once the effort has been made to develop ethics content in this way, it can easily be "lifted" from a curriculum and offered in the field to practicing professionals who did not have ethics education included in their formal nursing program. This last point is important, for as Aroskar has pointed out, ethics content is neither readily available nor usually required in nursing programs throughout this country.[15]

One final comment regarding methodology. Because ethics, by its very nature, is frustrating and because health professionals generally appear to be motivated to search for "the" answer, to concretize, the learner's initial contact with ethics should be in the form of a concrete problem. The educator should try presenting an actual practice situation or case to the learners and then ask the classic question, what should you do? This approach is an excellent attention getter. In addition, it clearly demonstrates the practice implications and reality orientation of ethics. Finally, it can help learners to identify what they do not know and help motivate them to want to know.

•   •   •

Clearly, there is a need for ethics content to be included in nursing curricula. We have gone beyond the why of ethics education. It is now time to consider the what and the how. The sooner these aspects are analyzed, the sooner we can get on with the teaching of ethics.

REFERENCES

1. Aroskar, M. "Ethics in the Nursing Curriculum." *Nursing Outlook* 25 (April 1977) p. 260-264.
2. Brody, H. *Ethical Decisions in Medicine* 2nd ed. (Boston: Little, Brown 1981) p. 18.
3. Ibid. p. 84.
4. Frankena, W.K. "Toward a Philosophy of Moral Education" in Scheffler, I., ed. *Philosophy and Education: Modern Readings* 2nd ed. (Boston: Allyn and Bacon 1966) p. 230.
5. Callahan, D. and Bok, S., eds. *Ethics Teaching in Higher Education* (New York: Plenum Press 1980) p. 61-80.

6. Brody. *Ethical Decisions in Medicine.*

7. Thompson, J.B. and Thompson, H.O. *Ethics in Nursing* (New York, Macmillan 1981).

8. Fromer, M.J. *Ethical Issues in Healthcare* (St. Louis, Mo.: C.V. Mosby 1981).

9. Frankena, W.K. *Ethics* 2nd ed. (Englewood, N.J.: Prentice-Hall 1973).

10. Smart, J.J.C. and Williams, B. *Utilitarianism For and Against* (Cambridge: Cambridge University Press 1973).

11. Kant, I. *Groundwork of the Metaphysics of Morals* 3rd ed. (New York: Harper and Row 1965).

12. Reich, W.T., ed. *Encyclopedia of Bioethics* (New York: Free Press 1978).

13. Zajonc, R.B. and Markus, G.B. "Birth Order and Intellectual Development." *Psychological Review* 82 (January 1975) p. 74–88.

14. Gilbert, C. "Ethics and Its Application to Nursing: An Experimental Study with Baccalaureate Nursing Students Utilizing an Engineering Design with a Specific Learning Program." Doctoral diss., University of Michigan, 1980 (Microfilm 1-178).

15. Aroskar. "Ethics in the Nursing Curriculum."

An Educational Strategy for Enhancement of Moral–Ethical Decision Making

Elizabeth O. Bridston, Ed.D., R.N.
Assistant Professor
Division of Nursing
New York University
New York, New York

BACCALAUREATE nursing program's have traditionally specified two kinds of educational goals, cognitive and affective.[1] A problem that teachers face in planning undergraduate nursing curricula is to adequately provide for learning in both areas. The majority of instructional objectives written for nursing courses are cognitive, that is, they identify knowledge, understanding and skills to be achieved in specific subject matter content areas. These are to be demonstrated by performance, or through specific observable and measurable behavior, usually assessed by criterion-referenced tests.

More general educational goals, however, prescribe attainments of certain kinds of beliefs, attitudes, values and principles upon which students are expected to base their judgments and decisions in the practice of their profession. Because attainment of these goals in the affective domain is so much more difficult to observe, measure and assess, pursuit of such aims is generally given relatively less attention in planning curricula and instructional strategies for nursing education programs.

The teaching strategy to be described here has an objective measure. At the same time it contributes to an affective goal: the enhancement of nursing student competency in decision making when facing moral-ethical dilemmas in clinical practice. It is hoped that it fosters the development of cognitive development and moral reasoning based on commitment to moral and ethical values derived from universal principles.

EDUCATIONAL PREPARATION FOR MORAL-ETHICAL DECISION MAKING

Giving nursing care to clients in any setting inevitably draws the student into problem situations or dilemmas that demand decision making on the part of the nursing student. Teachers who hold post-clinical conferences can identify any number of such problems that students face in clinical settings. There is little doubt that nursing programs excel in preparing and measuring objectives for the knowledge and skills needed in clinical practice. But are these objectives integrally related to preparation for moral-ethical decision making?

This question led me to hold dilemma discussion seminars where each student presented a dilemma that was drawn from

Are nursing program objectives integrally related to preparation for moral-ethical decision making?

clinical practice. Theoretical content in nursing and other sciences was related to the situation and discussed thoroughly in the seminars. The discussions always included a format that focused on the dilemma and on the reasoning or thinking of each student as the decision was made. Also, the procedure provided for a corporate analysis with peers of the individual's reasoning leading to the decision. Although it might be considered potentially threatening for a student to be subjected to this kind of scrutiny, the fact is that over the period of a year almost all students responded positively to planned dilemma discussions with peers.

During the academic year 1980-1981 a dilemma discussion with junior-level nursing students was held each week in a course on maternity nursing. Students were exposed to ethical-moral issues as they participated in the weekly dilemma discussions. This involved practice in facing real-life problem situations or dilemmas. Tension was evident as students struggled to make a decision and to explain their reasoning for the choice to peers. This tension probably indicates concern and conflict; it also shows involvement in the issues and in the particular client situation. As students shared and discussed the basis for their decisions in particular dilemmas and were exposed to peer reasoning that was different from their own, there was evidence that students changed the basis of their reasoning, that there was growth.

This growth was measured objectively through the use of the Defining Issues Test (DIT), which was given as a pretest and posttest each semester. This test measures the percent of responses at the level of principled moral reasoning, the postconventional level. The score is the P score, the percent of responses in this category. Kohlberg's schema of six stages and three levels of moral development is the model for the DIT.

The preconventional level includes stages one and two—orientation toward punishment and orientation toward satisfaction of self. The conventional level includes stages three and four—conformity to stereotypical images of good behavior and conformity to rules of law and order. The postconventional level includes stages five and six—conformity to agreed upon social contract and acceptance of universal principles such as justice, equality, empathy and dignity. The level of principled reasoning and any change in the *P* score during the semester were measured objectively by the DIT. At the same time, the enhancement of moral–ethical decision making was also observed in a subjective way through student reports.

The educational strategy of planned dilemma discussions is one way to bridge the gap between classroom teaching of knowledge and skills and the practice of nursing. This strategy is directed toward student growth not precisely measured by written tests or observed behavior. It is, rather, focused on student growth which can be identified by student self-evaluation related to specific objectives. Student responses to specific objectives, which are reported below, would be considered subjective data. They refer to values and beliefs and, therefore, are within the affective domain.

Nurses collect this type of data from clients in health assessments. What clients feel, think, favor or reject is a part of all nursing care plans. Just as client-reported data are a significant part of a health assessment, so student-reported learning

and areas of growth would seem to be part of a holistic approach to teaching. As students learn to recognize their own levels of reasoning and those of their peers, so they are able to do so with clients. This ability can be seen when the nurse recognizes the stage of reasoning or thinking used by a client. It helps a client when the nurse accepts stage-two decision making (concern for self and self alone) rather than demanding stage-four decisions (following prescribed behavior) which the client unwillingly accepts. The theoretical basis for using this model of Kohlberg's six stages of moral development supports this point of view.

THEORETICAL BASIS FOR THE EDUCATIONAL STRATEGY OF DILEMMA DISCUSSIONS

Dewey asserted that all individuals go through stages of moral development and that movement through these stages can be enhanced by stimulating the problem-solving and decision-making capabilities during the years of formal education.[2] Kohlberg, building on Piaget's stages of cognitive development, posits six stages of moral development.[3] These theorists propose that there are distinct, sequential developmental stages that are the same for all individuals. Interaction with the environment is assumed to be fundamental in this process of moral developmental growth from one stage to the next. Specifically, discussion of situations that involve conflict over moral issues and actions to be taken means that there is exposure to group members' reasoning which in turn motivates progress through successive stages.

Kohlberg advocates the fostering of principled moral reasoning (postconventional or stages five and six) as an educational goal. However, he does not believe that moral reasoning can be taught directly. As physiological and cognitive developmental processes are advanced through interactions between the individual and the environment, moral development progresses as the individual grows and goes to school. Kohlberg and Gilligan emphasize that "School experience must represent real life experience in stimulating development."[4]

But how can real-life experience be brought into the classroom? One means takes the form of a dilemma or problem situation taken from the nursing student's actual practice. Within the context of such a dynamic interchange students' potential for growth would seem to increase. As Kohlberg and Turiel describe it, "An individual cannot be taught stage five principles directly because he must generate them himself; the task of the teacher is to facilitate such a process."[5] The educational strategy of dilemma discussions described in this article is a means of providing teachers in clinical settings with a strategy for facilitating moral development and providing student nurses with a self-generating process of growth in moral development.

STRATEGY FOR SELF-ENHANCEMENT OF MORAL DEVELOPMENT

The educational strategy for self-enhancement of moral development can be described as having a traditional theoretical model as a base with the integration of the holistic concept of student self-

responsibility to promote moral development. Students draw from their own experience for their seminar presentations. There is a two-hour seminar each week composed of no more than ten nursing students and their clinical instructor. In this way all the participants are in the same area of practice. In the study discussed here, the students were in agencies serving the childbearing family. Theoretical content in biological, social and nursing science is part of each case discussion. This means that classroom theoretical content and clinical knowledge and skills are part of the dilemma discussion.

The dilemma discussion itself is structured using Galbraith's and Jones's model based on experience with dilemma discussions in high school science classes.[6] The format includes four steps:

1. confronting a moral dilemma;
2. stating a position on the dilemma;
3. testing one's reasoning for the decision; and
4. reflecting on one's reasoning and that of one's peers.

The discussions are moderated by the clinical instructor, who facilitates the process by such devices as focusing upon the predecision reasoning, contrasting and comparing different reasoning or thinking stated by group members and drawing out students to help them clarify their reasoning. The format may include analysis by the instructor of the characteristics of this reasoning so that students are aware of the concepts and presuppositions from which their decisions have arisen.

The purpose of this type of dilemma discussion, with the focus on the individual's own reasoning, is to draw students into looking more closely at the basis for their decision making and to be exposed to the

> *The purpose of dilemma discussion, with the focus on the individual's own reasoning, is to draw students into looking more closely at the basis for their decision making.*

critical reasoning of their peers. As they are involved in a dilemma debate, the tension increases; in the process of deciding between or among several difficult alternate choices, students may open themselves to considering other bases for decision making.

As Galbraith and Jones explain, "Students who participate regularly in discussions of moral dilemmas often begin to articulate reasoning at higher stages of development. This evidence indicates that exchanging reasoning during a group discussion of a moral dilemma can stimulate moral development through the stages."[7] The closer the dilemma is to real life, the more clearly students state their reasoning. Role playing is one way to approximate reality or real life. Kohlberg explains, "Moral judgment is based on sympathy for others."[8] There may be student-planned or spontaneous role playing initiated by the instructor to bring the reality of the situation to the seminar, to heighten the tension and to involve the students more personally.

OTHER RESEARCH DEFINES THE PROBLEM

Nonnursing intervention studies

There have been few reported studies using an intervention to enhance the level of principled reasoning in college students.

The first research using dilemma discussions as an intervention was described by Blatt and Kohlberg.[9] The participants were not college level but boys, aged 11 to 12 in one group and 11 to 16 in another. After dilemma discussions the experimental group showed progress toward principled reasoning when compared to the control group.

This type of study has since been replicated by Blatt and Kohlberg, with positive results, using the interview technique of measurement designed by Kohlberg to define the results. It can be concluded that these initial studies in the field have shown that moral dilemma discussions facilitate progress toward principled reasoning. The researchers state, "While formal moral education has been a subject of thoughtful concern since the time of Socrates, the present study is the first research report of a substantial and relatively enduring effect of a formal program of moral education upon children."[10] This research was the first intervention study in the field of moral development.

Rest reported the results of testing 136 samples which contained a total of 5,714 subjects.[11] He summarized the data and showed that the hypothetical relation between the *P* score, the measure of moral reasoning and the educational level ranged from junior high subjects with DIT *P* scores of 20 to 30 percent, to senior high subjects at 31 to 40 percent, to college subjects at 41 to 50 percent, to graduate subjects with 51 to 60 percent, and to doctoral subjects between 61 and 70 percent. Rest concluded that the theoretical implications of the findings from the many studies that have been conducted using the DIT and *P* score as a measure of moral reasoning lent support "to the DIT as an assessment instrument and to the cognitive developmental approach of studying morality."[12]

The DIT has been used as a pretest and a posttest following an intervention to measure change in stage level. Rest listed only 16 studies using the DIT in this way.[13] Among these 16 studies only 6 recorded samples from college-level students. All these intervention studies (as described by Rest in 1979) were conducted by non-nurses. Of the six researchers, three reported significant changes in P scores after an intervention and three found no significant changes. Since that time two nursing intervention research studies have been reported, which will be presented later in this article.

Panowitsch, in a study of junior college students, found that after an ethics course subjects ($N = 152$) gained on the P score as compared to those who were not in this class and that there was a significant difference in posttest P scores.[14] In a similar study (as reported by Rest), Piwko studied college students and found that after ten two-hour sessions on moral values and commitments, there were gains in the subjects' ($N = 68$) posttest P scores.[15] Likewise, Whitely and Nelson found that college freshmen ($N = 77$), after an eight-month course in psychological growth, made gains in their posttest P scores.[16] However, it should be noted that a number of investigators have reported nonsignificant gains in moral reasoning following various forms and periods of interventions through a course or module.[17-19]

Nursing intervention studies

Two nurse researchers, including me, have subsequently reported on research using an intervention to enhance moral reasoning. The DIT was used as a measure in both studies. In the first, St. Denis included nursing student volunteers from two baccalaureate nursing programs and a master of science nursing program.[20] Data from the three programs were pooled for analysis. One of the interventions was a moral education strategy. Participants exposed to this strategy were found to have significant changes in their posttest P scores.

I studied 69 freshman-level baccalaureate nursing students.[21] The intervention consisted of seven 30-minute dilemma discussions over a period of a semester for the experimental group and a seminar for the control group. This pattern was repeated in a second semester. In each semester the experimental group had a positive change from pretest to posttest on the P scores. This change from pretest to posttest was not statistically significant in either semester.

This research has been continued with junior-level baccalaureate nursing students ($N = 42$) with no control group.[22] After one year of a two-year study, which is still in progress, I found definite positive changes in P scores from pretest to posttest, although these, technically, lacked statistical significance. Student evaluation forms written by participants at the end of each semester indicated a positive response. For example, for items rated as high, moderate or low, student response as to the value of dilemma discussions for raising "level of consciousness regarding moral–ethical issues," was 75 percent in the high rating and 25 percent in the moderate rating. In "group leading skills increase," 53 percent chose the high rating and 44 percent the moderate one. In "level of group interaction," 72 percent selected the high category and 26 percent the moderate rating. In each of the above, 97 to 98 percent of the group members of the dilemma discussions responded in the high to moderate ratings.

These results might indicate growth in important areas such as awareness and recognition of ethical dimensions in the students' environments. If this is true, a great gain may have been attained in meeting goals in the affective domain. These goals, which are directed toward the generation of certain attitudes, values and principles within students, remain an elusive task for educators in terms of precise measurement. However, this should not inhibit the pursuit of such critical goals.

A HOLISTIC APPROACH TO MORAL DEVELOPMENT

The theory of moral development and the use of an intervention to influence this process of growth may seem to be atomistic rather than holistic insofar as the theory describes separate, mutually exclusive stages. This may appear to be incompatible with a continuum of growth and moral development. Nevertheless, although human beings are whole and unified, the use of this model in which various levels of reasoning are delineated is one way of better understanding human moral reasoning. For example, Rest and his colleagues resisted labeling individuals at one stage or another. They were interested in classifying development by use of a continuous variable rather than stage typing by subject.[23] Within a holistic framework it can be said that individuals utilize all stages.

Another researcher who used the DIT as a measure discussed the nature of developmental status and progress. "To characterize subjects as stage 1, 2, 3, 4, 5, or 6 ... distorts the data, since it represents a person's actual moral-judgment behavior. The emergence of conventional morality is not an 'all' or 'none' affair but rather a sequence of small presumably numerous transitions."[24]

Measurement of the level of moral developmental stage change, therefore, reflects movement which is gradual and difficult to measure. The P score is interpreted within such a context. By using group norms of P scores, teachers can see if their classes are within the range for that educational level. Group rather than individual scores may then indicate several aspects of moral development during the college years. These scores may show moral developmental status compared to other baccalaureate nursing students or general college students. Or, from another angle, these comparative scores may reveal growth or lack of growth from one period to another, or particular growth after a period of interventions.

Comparisons can also be made among nurses who are practicing in various fields. These comparisons have become possible recently through the research of Crisham,[25] Ketefian,[26] Munhall,[27] Murphy,[28] Schleicher,[29] Schoenrock,[30] St. Denis,[31] and myself.[32] These studies, among others using the DIT as a measure, contribute to and support the theory of moral development as a continuum. They provide evidence that there are levels of moral reasoning and that principled moral reasoning increases as the level of education advances.

Within the context of the theory of moral development, the dilemma discus-

> *Through the practice of facing moral–ethical issues with peers, individual students' consciousness of their own and their peers' reasoning and thinking is heightened.*

sion strategy, as an intervention, has potential for enhancing several aspects of moral development. Through the practice of facing moral-ethical issues with peers, individual students' consciousness of their own and their peers' reasoning and thinking which precedes decision making is heightened.

Furthermore, awareness and sensitivity to these issues as they exist in nurse–client situations increase. This leads to an ability to perceive the reasoning of clients as they struggle with decision making in dilemma situations. As a result, nursing students increasingly become facilitators for clients. An openended holistic process is set in motion: students' moral sensibilities are heightened by a training and educational program involving patient care and the dilemmas arising out of that practice. And this in turn prepares them, as eventual professionals, to facilitate and support their clients' own moral decision-making process.

REFERENCES

1. Krathwohl, D.R., Bloom, B.S. and Masis, B.B. *Taxonomy of Educational Objectives, Handbook II: Affective Domain* (New York: David McKay 1964).
2. Dewey, J. *Moral Principles in Education* (Boston: Houghton Mifflin Co. 1909).
3. Kohlberg, L. "Stage and Sequence: The Cognitive-Developmental Approach to Socialization" in D.A. Goslin, ed. *Handbook of Socialization Theory and Research* (Chicago: Rand McNally 1969) p. 347-355.
4. Kohlberg, L. and Gilligan, C. "The Adolescent as a Philosopher: The Discovery of the Self in a Postconventional World." *Daedalus* 100 (Fall 1971) p. 1083.
5. Kohlberg, L. and Turiel, E. "Moral Development and Moral Education" in Lesser, G., ed. *Psychology and Educational Practice* (Glenview, Ill.: Scott Foresman 1971) p. 410-465.
6. Galbraith, R.E. and Jones, T.M. "Teaching Strategies for Moral Dilemmas, An Application of Kohlberg's Theory of Moral Development to the Social Studies Classroom." *Social Education* 39:6 (1975) p. 19.
7. Ibid. p. 18.
8. Kohlberg, L. "From Is to Ought: How to Commit the Naturalistic Fallacy and Get Away with It in the Study of Moral Development" in Mischel, T., ed. *Cognitive Development and Epistemology* (New York: Academic Press 1971) p. 190.
9. Blatt, M.M. and Kohlberg, L. "The Effects of Classroom Moral Discussion upon Children's Level of Moral Judgment" in Kohlberg, L. and Turiel, E. eds.

Recent Research In Moral Development (New York: Holt, Rinehart and Winston 1973) p. 49-52.
10. Ibid.
11. Rest, J. *Moral Judgment Related to Sample Characteristics.* Report to National Institute of Mental Health Grant # 8703 MH 24988 (Minneapolis: University of Minnesota 1976).
12. Ibid. p. 24.
13. Rest, J. *Development in Judging Moral Issues* (Minneapolis: University of Minnesota Press 1979).
14. Panowitsch, H.R. "Change and Stability in the Defining Issues Test (DIT); An Objective Measure of Moral Development." *Dissertation Abstracts International* 37:1 (1979) p. 201-A.
15. Rest, J. *Development in Judging Moral Issues.* p. 212-213.
16. Ibid.
17. Ibid.
18. Ibid.
19. Ibid.
20. St. Denis, H. "Effects of Moral Education Strategies on Nursing Students Moral Reasoning and Level of Self-Actualization." Ph.D. dissertation, Catholic University, 1980.
21. Bridston, E.O. "The Development of Principled Moral Reasoning in Baccalaureate Nursing Students." *Dissertation Abstracts International* 40:3 (1979) p. 1237-A.
22. Bridston, E.O. *The Use of Moral Dilemma Discussions*

in *Educating Nurses for Care of the Childbearing Family*. Report for Nursing Research Emphasis Grants for Doctoral Programs in Nursing, DHHS, HRA, Division of Nursing, Grant 1R21 NU-00833-01, (Hyattsville, Md.: DHHS 1980-1981).

23. Rest, J. et al. "Judging the Important Issues in Moral Dilemmas—An Objective Measure of Development." *Developmental Psychology* 11:6 (1975) p. 738-748.

24. Moir, J. "Egocentrism and the Emergence of Conventional Morality in Preadolescent Girls." *Child Development* 45:2 (1974) p. 303.

25. Crisham, P. "Measuring Moral Judgment in Nursing Dilemmas." *Nursing Research* 30:2 (1981) p. 104-110.

26. Ketefian, S. "Critical Thinking, Educational Preparation and Development of Moral Judgment among Selected Groups of Practicing Nurses." *Nursing Research* 30:2 (1981) p. 171-175.

27. Munhall, P. "Moral Reasoning Levels of Nursing Students and Faculty in a Baccalaureate Nursing Program." *Image* 12:3 (1980) p. 57-61.

28. Murphy, C.P. "Levels of Moral Reasoning in a Selected Group of Nurse Practitioners." *Dissertation Abstracts International* 38:2 (1976) p. 953-B.

29. Schleicher, M. "Moral Judgments: A Study Investigating Instrument Development for the Nursing Profession." Ph.D. dissertation, University of Michigan, 1978.

30. Schoenrock, N.B. "An Analysis of Moral Reasoning Levels and the Implications for Nursing Curriculum." *Dissertation Abstracts International* 39:3 (1979) p. 4035-A.

31. St. Denis, H. "Effects of Moral Education Strategies on Nursing Students Moral Reasoning and Level of Self-Actualization."

32. Bridston, E.O. "The Development of Principled Moral Reasoning in Baccalaureate Nursing Students."

Index